What Are We FEEDING OUR KIDS?

What Are We
FEEDING
OUR KIDS?

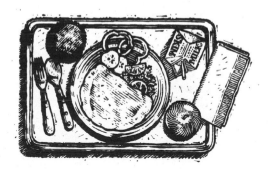

MICHAEL F. JACOBSON PH.D.

*EXECUTIVE DIRECTOR, CENTER FOR SCIENCE
IN THE PUBLIC INTEREST*

& BRUCE MAXWELL

WORKMAN PUBLISHING, NEW YORK

Library of Congress Cataloging-in-Publication Data
Jacobson, Michael F.
What are we feeding our kids? / by Michael F. Jacobson and Bruce Maxwell
p. cm.
ISBN 1-56305-101-X
1. Children—Nutrition. 2. Children—Nutrition—Psychological aspects.
3. Junk food. I. Maxwell, Bruce. II. Title.
RJ206.J28 1994
613.2'083—dc20   94-934
                    CIP

Cover illustration by Greg King
Cover Photograph by Mary Bloom

Workman books are available at a special discount when purchased in bulk
for special premiums and sales promotions as well as for fund-raising or educational use. Special editions or book excerpts can also be created to specifica-
tion. For details, contact the Special Sales Director at the address below.

Workman Publishing Company, Inc.
708 Broadway
New York, NY 10003

Manufactured in the United States of America

First printing August 1994
10 9 8 7 6 5 4 3 2 1

To Sonya Jeanette, the light of my life, who is providing a reality test of all the advice in this book. — M.F.J.

For Barbara — B.M.

Acknowledgments

W e'd like to thank the hundreds of doctors, social scientists, school food service directors, citizen activists, government and corporate spokespersons, and parents who kindly agreed to be interviewed for this book. We are grateful to our colleagues at the Center for Science in the Public Interest for the work they have done over the years that contributed to this book. Bonnie Liebman, CSPI's director of nutrition and a mother of three, deserves special thanks for carefully reading the entire manuscript and providing always prescient comments. She also contributed to numerous sections, especially those about fat, heart disease, and cancer. Jayne Hurley, CSPI's expert on nutritional values of natural and processed foods, helped compile figures on sodium, fat, and sugar and develop CSPI's Healthy Eating Pyramid. Other CSPI staffers who worked on children's nutrition and food safety issues include Jennifer Douglas, David Schardt, Bruce Silverglade, Ingrid VanTuinen, Geoffrey Barron, and Lisa Lefferts. William G. Crook, M.D., offered constructive suggestions regarding food sensitivities. Finally, we would like to acknowledge the thoughtful and expert editing by Suzanne Rafer and Margot Herrera, and the assistance of Shannon Ryan at Workman Publishing.

Contents

Preface

Over the course of twenty years in the United States Senate, I have fought to improve the nutritional health of children. I have campaigned to expand the Special Supplemental Nutrition Program for Women, Infants and Children; to reach more hungry children through the school breakfast and summer food programs; and to improve the nutritional quality of all school meals.

Twenty-five million children eat federally subsidized school lunches every day. Those meals should provide all the nutrients children need to grow and to learn. I have pushed legislation to require that school meals include less fat and more fresh fruits and vegetables. And I have fought to keep vending machines out of schools.

What Are We Feeding Our Kids? will be a powerful tool in the battle to improve the health of our nation's children. Michael Jacobson and Bruce Maxwell have done a great job of translating the latest scientific knowledge about healthy eating into practical steps that parents can take.

Children ages 4 to 12 influence more than $128 billion in family spending each year, and much of it is spent on snacks and junk food. It's no wonder given the amount of television advertising for these products directed at children.

But the junk food purveyors have met their match in Michael Jacobson and Bruce Maxwell. Every parent should read *What Are We Feeding Our Kids?* This book warns about misleading TV commercials and shows parents how they can protect their children's health through better nutrition.

What Are We Feeding Our Kids? should also be required reading for all those in Congress and throughout the United

States who are interested in health care reform. With all the talk about controlling skyrocketing health care costs, we need to remember that an ounce of prevention is indeed worth a pound of cure. And proper nutrition is the cornerstone of prevention.

Real reform of the health care system must begin with our children. Teaching them to eat right — teaching them the link between good nutrition and good health — is a lesson they will carry with them for the rest of their lives.

—Senator Patrick J. Leahy
July 28, 1994

Feeding Our Kids Right— What Could Be More Important?

I t's an idyllic morning as the commercial opens. A blond, pony-tailed girl practices hurdles in the farmyard. She clears the first barrier, but her foot catches on the second and she falls flat.

"I'll never be ready for the trials tomorrow," she moans to Tony the Tiger, who's coaching.

"We'll try again after a complete breakfast including my vitamin-packed Frosted Flakes," says Tony. "They bring out the tiger in you!" They sit at a picnic table for breakfast, which includes Frosted Flakes, milk, orange juice, and a muffin. Two words pop up over the picture: "Vitamin packed."

Enter her obnoxious little brother, who's on his way to school. "She won't make it," he sneers. "She's no good."

The girl returns to practicing; the scene dissolves into the next day's race. As she runs, the theme song blares: "Show 'em you're a tiger, show 'em what you can do. The taste of Tony's Frosted Flakes brings out the tiger in you!" With Tony and her brother cheering her on, she wins the race.

It's an all-American morality play, 30 seconds of sugar-coated goo designed to sell sugar-coated goop. The ad is full of subtly deceptive messages, targeted separately at children and their parents.

To an impressionable child, the ad's message is clear: Eating Frosted Flakes will make you a sports star. As an added bonus, it also will transform your little brother from a brat into a hero-worshiper. If only life were so simple.

To a parent who may be watching, the message is equally clear: This "vitamin-packed" cereal is nutritious. While it's true that Kellogg fortifies the cereal with vitamins and iron, fortification is largely a marketing gimmick designed to placate parents worried about buying sugary goop.

Calling Frosted Flakes "sugary goop" isn't hyperbole: The cereal is 39 percent sugar. A one-ounce serving, or about three-quarters of a cup, has nearly three teaspoons of sugar. Until a few years ago, Kellogg called the cereal "Sugar Frosted Flakes." In response to parents' growing concerns about their children's sugar intake, Kellogg quietly dropped "Sugar" from the name. Unfortunately, it didn't bother to lower the sugar content.

Other companies are equally sneaky. General Foods changed "Super Sugar Crisp" to "Super Golden Crisp," but it didn't bother to lower the sugar level either. Faced with a choice of misleading consumers or making constructive, healthful changes in their products, food manufacturers all too often choose the flimflam. That's especially true today with foods they target at children.

Why is deception popular? Because it has worked so well for

so long. Phony health claims for foods date back at least a century. In the old days, marketers directed their deceptive claims at parents. But today, companies use television as an electronic salesman that beams messages directly to kids.

Of course, most food commercials aimed at children don't make nutrition claims. They instead seek to dazzle kids with flashy graphics, catchy tunes, and the unmistakable message that eating the food is fun, fun, fun. Almost invariably, the ads push foods loaded with fat, cholesterol, sodium, or sugar. For some reason, broccoli producers have never managed to create a good jingle for kids.

That's unfortunate, because there's evidence that what we eat as kids affects our later risk of disease and premature death, four of the seven leading killers of Americans are associated with our diet. They include heart disease, some types of cancer, stroke, and diabetes. Poor diets also may promote obesity, which often begins in childhood. Rates of childhood obesity have soared in recent years.

The Diet–Disease Connection

The Surgeon General of the United States, the American Heart Association, the National Cancer Institute, and other health agencies have urged that both kids and adults switch to heart-healthy diets. People today who ignore the growing evidence linking diet to serious health problems are like those in the late 1950s who pooh-poohed studies linking smoking to lung cancer.

Dr. Ernst Wynder, president of the American Health Foundation in New York City and one of the first researchers to link cigarette smoking to lung cancer, admits that although it's far easier to prove a relationship between smoking and lung cancer than between diet and disease, the evidence linking diet to disease is "almost as persuasive." Today, he's in the forefront of efforts to get children to eat healthy diets.

So, is there enough evidence to justify changing your children's diets? You bet. Research into the connection between children's diets and adult disease only started in earnest in the late 1970s and early 1980s, but researchers constantly are publishing new findings. Although they're years away from answering some questions and may never resolve others, it makes little sense to wait until they answer every question. The earlier you start your children on the road to good nutrition, the likelier they are to adopt healthy eating habits that will last throughout their lifetimes.

These needed dietary changes don't require turning your children's diets totally upside down. A variety of modest adjustments, taken together, can make a big difference. And you don't necessarily have to bar your children from ever again having a Big Mac, fries, and a Coke. Instead, you need to help them understand how they can occasionally fit those foods into a diet that is healthy overall.

So what constitutes a healthy diet for children? There used to be lots of conflicting answers to that question. No more. Today, the nation's leading health authorities agree on the general principles, even while they continue debating the details. Here's a quick summary of what kids age 2 or older should eat. (Please note that this diet isn't appropriate for children under age 2. We'll make recommendations for the youngest children in Chapter 10.) Kids should:

- Get no more than 25 to 30 percent of their calories from all types of fat, and less than 10 percent—ideally closer to 7 percent—of their calories from saturated fat.
- Limit their daily cholesterol intake to between 200 and 300 milligrams.

- Limit their daily sodium intake to a maximum of 2,400 milligrams, and preferably aim for a target of 1,800 milligrams.
- Limit their intake of refined sugar.
- Eat lots of foods rich in complex carbohydrates such as potatoes, pasta, beans, and whole-grain bread and cereal.
- Eat at least five servings of fresh fruits and vegetables every day.

Will eating this diet guarantee that your children won't ever develop diet-related diseases? No, it won't. Will it lower their risk of developing such diseases? Absolutely. It's like buckling your children into safety seats or seat belts when they ride in the car with you. If you get into an accident, being buckled in doesn't guarantee that your children will escape serious injury. But it does significantly lower their risk. If you're like most parents, that's enough to prompt you to make sure your children are always buckled in. Likewise, the opportunity to lower health risk should also spur you to make sure your children eat a healthy diet.

Why It's Important to Start Early

Some parents contend that children don't need to eat properly because they can always change their diet when they're older. Dr. Richard Garcia, a pediatrician who co-directs the Cleveland Clinic's program on fats in children's blood, has little patience for such arguments. "That has about the same kind of validity as saying it's okay for kids to smoke until they're 21—they can always quit," he said. "Or they can go ahead and get fat—they can always lose weight. Or they can forgo exercise—they can always take up an exercise program later on. That just doesn't make a lot of sense. Behaviors tend to be perpetuated. And it's awfully difficult to get rid of a behavior once it's a part of you."

Of course, eating a healthy diet is only one component—albeit a critical one—of a healthy lifestyle that minimizes the risk of disease. Your children also need to get lots of exercise, avoid obesity, and stay away from alcohol, tobacco, and drugs. Some of those healthy habits may be interrelated. For example, children who learn to take care of their bodies by eating healthy foods and exercising may be less inclined to smoke cigarettes or engage in other unhealthy activities.

What Kids Eat

If parents followed their children around, they might be shocked at their eating habits. Consider a 10-year-old girl living in the inner city of Washington, D.C., whom researchers from Georgetown University monitored for a whole day.[1] Her breakfast at home consisted of sugar-coated corn flakes, whole milk, a third of a can of Coke, and a chocolate brownie. While walking to school, she shared a bag of corn chips with a friend. For lunch at school, she ate most of a hamburger and a half pint of whole milk, only the corn from her mixed vegetables, a cupcake, part of a candy bar, and several gulps of Coke.

At a mid-afternoon class party, she ate a large piece of white cake with chocolate frosting, three handfuls of barbecue-flavored potato chips, peanuts, fruit punch, half of an imitation fruit roll, and two chocolate-covered peppermint candies.

While walking home, she bought a piece of apple pie and a can of Coke to share with a friend, ate a package of Reese's Pieces, and bought bubble gum to chew later. After arriving home, she got more money and returned to the store to buy a bag of potato chips to share with friends at the playground, who gave her orange soda in return. Only 90 minutes later, she ate all the dinner provided by the local recreation center: fried chicken breast, cole slaw, an orange, chocolate cookies, and fruit punch.

Back home at 6 P.M., she ate a fried fish stick from her parents' meal, four vanilla cookies, and five handfuls of popcorn, washing it all down with half a can of soda and a big glass of iced tea. And just before bedtime, she ate a banana and drank more iced tea.

That girl's diet may not be typical, but it illustrates several important trends in children's eating habits today:

• **Increased snacking.** Kids today are eating more snacks than ever before.[2] For many children, snacks provide more calories than any single meal during the day.

A study of 10-year-olds found that the average child got one-third of his or her calories from snacks, which commonly are high in fat, sugar, or sodium and low in vitamins and minerals. Nearly one in seven of the 10-year-olds got 50 percent to 70 percent of his or her calories from snacks. Some of the youngsters seemed to snack virtually hourly.[3] Many studies show that kids are more likely to snack heavily during sedentary activities like watching television.

Snacking itself isn't bad. Because they have small stomachs, many children can't eat at regular meals all the food they need to keep their bodies running and growing. For them, snacks are essential to getting adequate calories and nutrients. The key is avoiding unhealthy snacks like potato chips and soda and choosing healthy ones like bananas and fruit juice.

• **Increased eating away from home.** Kids and their families are eating out more than ever before. In 1992, the average American family spent 40 cents of every food dollar on snacks and meals eaten away from home, up from just 29 cents in 1970.[4] If that trend continues, in just a few years Americans will spend more money on meals eaten away from home than on food they cook themselves.

The nutritional quality of children's diets decreases the more

Ten of the Worst Children's Foods

- Soda pop
- Hamburgers
- Hot dogs
- Whole milk
- American cheese
- French fries and Tater Tots

- Pizza loaded with meat and cheese
- Chocolate bars
- Ice cream
- Bologna

they eat away from home (except for school lunches). That's not surprising, considering that much of the food at fast-food restaurants, in vending machines, and at convenience stores is relatively unhealthful. A Cornell University study found that the more frequently people ages 13 to 21 ate away from home, the fewer nutrients they consumed.[5] And a study reported by the National Research Council (a branch of the National Academy of Sciences) found that children who ate away from home the most tended to consume the highest levels of fat, sugar, sodium, and calories.[6]

• **Growing child autonomy in making food choices.** Children today have lots of spending money and frequently spend it on food. James McNeal, a marketing professor at Texas A&M University, estimates that in 1989 alone, children ages 4 to 12 spent over $2 billion on snacks and sweets.

Making food choices is a key part of children's striving for independence, and today they have more opportunities to express their independence than ever before. For instance, when they return home from school—often to empty houses—kids are free to turn on the TV and help themselves to a snack of their choosing. Unfortunately, children—frequently prodded by slick ads and ubiquitous snacking opportunities—make lots of poor food choices. On any given day:

- Children ages 1 to 5 are as likely to drink soft drinks as orange juice.[7]
- Children ages 8 to 11 are more likely to eat pretzels, potato chips, or crackers than potatoes, rice, or pasta.[8]
- Adolescents ages 12 to 18 are more likely to eat cupcakes, cookies, popsicles, or candy than apples, bananas, grapes, or raisins.[9]

Why do kids eat so poorly? The answer is complex, but four reasons stand out:

- **Junk foods *taste* good.** From birth, humans prefer the taste of something sweet—it's the only taste preference we're born with. Thus, it's no surprise that very young children usually prefer cupcakes over spinach. With continued exposure, humans also can develop preferences for fat and salt. That makes it all the more important to start kids eating well early.
- **Kids are surrounded by poor influences.** The poor influ-

Ten of the Best Children's Foods

- Fresh fruit and vegetables—especially carrot sticks, cantaloupe, oranges, watermelon, strawberries
- Chicken breast or drumstick without skin or breading
- Cheerios, Wheaties, or other whole-grain, low-sugar cereals
- Skim or 1 percent milk
- Extra-lean ground beef (Healthy Choice) or vegetarian burgers (Gardenburgers or Green Giant Harvest Burgers)

- Low-fat hot dogs (meat or Yves Veggie Cuisine Fat-Free weiners or Lightlife Fat-Free Smart Dogs)
- Non-fat ice cream or frozen yogurt
- Fat-free corn chips or potato chips
- Seasoned air-popped popcorn
- Whole-wheat crackers or Small World Animal Grahams

ences start right at home, and we're not just referring to TV commercials. In a national poll of 5,000 third- through twelfth-graders sponsored by Kellogg, only 38 percent said other members of their families usually ate the proper foods. It's not surprising that only 34 percent of the kids said they frequently ate healthy foods.[10]

Of course, families aren't the only poor influences. Peers, vending machines, and even school meals also can push kids in the wrong direction. We'll have more to say about those influences in later chapters.

• **Kids are ill-informed about nutrition.** Most children report in national surveys that they're taught nutrition at school. Yet their answers to basic questions about nutrition show that, for whatever reason, the lessons aren't sinking in.

For example, Kellogg's survey found that nearly 40 percent of students didn't know about the benefits of eating a high-fiber diet. More than one in five thought they should avoid eating complex carbohydrates such as pasta, potatoes, and rice.[11] That presumably reflects the old myth that starchy foods are bad. In fact, modern dietary guidelines recommend that all Americans—including children—increase their consumption of complex carbohydrates.

Kids also aren't learning basic nutrition skills. A poll of 11,000 eighth- and tenth-graders sponsored by three public health groups found that 57 percent of students couldn't figure out from a cereal label what the main ingredient was. And almost half the kids, when given two labels listing sugar contents, couldn't tell which cereal had more sugar.[12]

• **Kids don't see the need to eat properly.** Among teens in high school, only one in three reports that nutrition is very important.[13] For them, hanging out with their friends, trying to survive school, and wrangling a date are far more important than keeping their arteries clean. After all, they're going to live forever, aren't they?

Kids don't see their friends keeling over from heart attacks after downing Big Macs, ice cream, or hot dogs so they don't see any harm in eating them. They may be vaguely aware that the saturated fat in those foods can clog arteries, but they figure there's plenty of time to clean up their diet before they're old enough for heart attacks. As we'll explain in Part 1 of this book, they're dead wrong because deadly diseases begin in childhood, but eating the *right* foods can protect your child's health. In Part 2, we'll look at the factors that influence what kids eat: everything from television commercials to school lunch programs. And in Part 3, we'll examine what you can do in your home and your community to help ensure that both your own kids and other kids eat healthy diets.

PART 1

Food and Your Child's Health

CHAPTER 1

Fat and Cholesterol

> 66 *I do not think junk food is too bad for you. It has sugar in it—so what? You need sugar in your diet. I know too much sugar is not too good for you, but just cut down on other kinds of sugary foods like fruits and vegetables. I like fast food a lot because it is cheaper and tastes good. I eat a lot of sugary foods and am average weight for my height. . . .* 99

—An eighth-grade boy in Newark, New York

The boy's misconceptions about diet are staggering—and dangerous. His nonsensical ideas about sugar are bad enough. Yet far worse, he either doesn't know or doesn't care that many sugary junk foods and fast foods, including cookies, ice cream, chocolate bars, burgers, pizza, and tacos, also contain lots of fat and cholesterol.

The fat and cholesterol—not the sugar—should be his top concern. The sugar may be harming his teeth, but the fat and cholesterol may already be causing changes in his arteries that represent the beginnings of heart disease, the top killer of Americans. The fat may also cause cancer later in life.

Efforts to limit children's consumption of fat and cholesterol are relatively new. Until recently, parents worried primarily about dietary *deficiencies*. They sought to protect their children

A Fast Look at Fat and Cholesterol

*T*o *understand the roles of various types of fat and cholesterol, it may help to know a few key terms:*

• **Total fat:** This term encompasses all types of dietary fats, including both saturated and unsaturated fats. Any fat-containing food contains saturated, monounsaturated, and polyunsaturated fatty acids, but one of those types usually predominates and determines the effect on health. Fats that are liquid at room temperature are called oils. Amounts of dietary fats are measured in grams.

• **Saturated fat:** Americans get most of their saturated fat from dairy products, meat, poultry, and vegetable shortening. Coconut oil, palm kernel oil, and palm oil are also high in saturated fat. Too much saturated fat in the diet can raise blood cholesterol levels. "Saturated" is a chemical term meaning that fats are fully saturated with hydrogen atoms.

• **Unsaturated fat:** There are two types of unsaturated fat: polyunsaturated and monounsaturated. The biggest sources of polyunsaturated fat are several kinds of oils—corn, cottonseed, safflower, soybean, and sunflower—along with some fish, tub margarines, mayonnaise, walnuts, almonds, and pecans. The biggest sources of monounsaturated fats are poultry, shortening, meat, and dairy products; olive and canola oils also contain high levels. The unsaturated fats generally do not raise blood cholesterol levels. The term "polyunsaturated" means that a molecule is missing four, six, or

from diseases such as rickets, pellagra, scurvy, beriberi, and goiter, all caused by a lack of certain vitamins and minerals.

Today, increasing affluence and the fortification of foods with vitamins and minerals have virtually eliminated those deficiency diseases in the United States and other developed countries. Unfortunately, diseases "of dietary excess and imbalance"

more hydrogen atoms; "monounsaturates" are missing two.

• **Partially hydrogenated vegetable oil:** To make vegetable oils harder and more stable, companies mix them with hydrogen. That increases the amount of saturated fat and also creates *trans* fats. *Trans* fats are monounsaturated but, unlike natural monounsaturated fat, they raise blood cholesterol levels. Thus, *trans* fats are at least as bad as saturated fats. The word *trans* refers to the three-dimensional shape of the molecules.

• **Dietary cholesterol:** This cholesterol, which is found in foods, is the same fatty substance that is found in human blood. Only foods of animal origin, such as eggs, meat, poultry, fish, and dairy products, contain dietary cholesterol. In many people, dietary cholesterol significantly boosts blood cholesterol levels. But in others it has little effect. Cholesterol is measured in milligrams.

• **Blood cholesterol:** Cholesterol occurs in everyone's blood. The body manufactures it, and more enters the body in the form of dietary cholesterol. High levels of blood cholesterol increase the risk of heart disease. Cholesterol travels in the blood in little packages of fat and protein called lipoproteins. Cholesterol in high-density lipoproteins (HDL cholesterol) is the "good" cholesterol; it is actually being carried out of the body. On the other hand, the cholesterol in low-density lipoproteins (LDL cholesterol) is the "bad" cholesterol; it is headed for your artery walls.

have replaced the old diseases of dietary deficiencies, according to *The Surgeon General's Report on Nutrition and Health,* which was published in 1988. Diseases linked to eating too much of the wrong foods "now rank among the leading causes of illness and death in the United States," the report said.[1]

There's no way to determine diet's exact role in any particular case of heart disease, cancer, or other disease. Cancer cells don't carry little signs proclaiming, "I grew because this person didn't eat enough vegetables." However, there's strong evidence that diet plays a critical role in many diseases suffered by millions of people. And while diet is not the only factor in disease development, it *is* one that you can control. You can't change your children's genetic makeup, and you can't totally alter their environment. But you can influence what your children eat and help them develop healthy attitudes toward food.

In this chapter, we'll primarily focus on how fat and cholesterol affect the risk of heart disease. We'll also look at the latest research linking fat with cancer.

Fat and Heart Disease

During the Korean War, U.S. Army pathologists examined the bodies of 300 American soldiers killed in battle to learn about wound ballistics. Almost by accident, they made a startling discovery: Arteries in most of the young men already showed signs of heart disease. More than three-quarters of the soldiers had significant evidence of atherosclerosis, or clogging of the arteries. Fatty deposits had narrowed the coronary arteries—the arteries that feed blood to the heart muscle—to half or less of their normal size in 15 percent of the soldiers. Their average age: 22.[2] (By contrast, the arteries of Asian soldiers were remarkably clear and healthy.)

Those findings stunned the medical community. Doctors had thought that heart disease only affected older adults. After all, heart attacks or strokes rarely occur before age 40. The Korean War findings confounded everything they knew—or thought they knew. Did heart disease actually begin sometime before adulthood? And what on earth was causing it to appear in such young men?

Nearly 20 years later, U.S. Army doctors conducted a nearly identical study of the hearts of 105 American soldiers killed in Vietnam. The results were strikingly similar to those from the Korean War. Nearly half the soldiers had some degree of atherosclerosis, and 5 percent had severe disease. Again, the soldiers' average age was 22.[3]

Today, research spurred partly by the studies of soldiers killed in Korea and Vietnam is finally answering some of the questions about the origins of heart disease. While much remains unknown, doctors agree on one thing: Heart disease begins in childhood.

Atherosclerosis begins as fatty streaks, which can appear in the arteries of children as young as age 3. Those streaks, composed of fat and cholesterol, penetrate the lining of the arterial wall. Fatty streaks can continue to spread during the teens, twenties, thirties, and later. The fatty streaks themselves don't cause problems, since they are flat and don't interfere with blood flow.

In most people, some fatty streaks fade away, others remain unchanged, and yet others progress into advanced lesions called fibrous plaques. It's still unclear why different streaks act in different ways.

The progression into fibrous plaques is the first sign of real trouble. These bulging plaques, which can start developing as early as the late teens, can eventually reduce or cut off blood flow.[4] "The real problem is not so much what causes fatty streaks, but what causes some of them to be transformed into fibrous plaques and other more advanced lesions in a person's twenties and thirties," said Dr. Henry McGill, Jr., a pioneer in research on the beginnings of heart disease who is the scientific director at the Southwest Foundation for Biomedical Research in San Antonio, Texas.

No one knows precisely what causes fatty streaks to spread,

some streaks to progress into plaques, or some plaques to grow faster than others. However, two studies have found that cholesterol levels in the blood correlate with the growth of streaks and plaques in children and young adults.

In the first study, Louisiana State University researchers examined thousands of children ages 2½ and above in Bogalusa, Louisiana. They looked for "risk factors"—behaviors and biological measurements known to affect *adults'* risk of heart disease. They took the children's blood pressure, checked whether the children smoked or were obese, and measured levels of cholesterol and other substances in their blood. Researchers examined some of the children several times during the study, which stretched from 1973 through the mid-1980s.[5]

Thirty-five of the children died during the study, either in accidents or from other causes. When they died, the researchers were allowed to conduct autopsies to measure fatty streaks and other lesions in their arteries.

For each person who died, the researchers matched the individual's risk-factor data while alive with his or her lesion measurements after death. The aim: to see whether any risk factor was linked to the extent of lesions in children.

The autopsies revealed a strong link between cholesterol levels in the blood and lesions. Those who had the highest levels of total cholesterol and LDL ("bad") cholesterol had the most fatty streaks. By contrast, those with the highest levels of HDL ("good") cholesterol had the fewest fatty streaks.

A second study, published in 1990 and known as PDAY (for Pathobiological Determinants of Atherosclerosis in Youth), confirmed the link between blood cholesterol levels and lesions in young people. In this study, researchers in eight communities around the United States collected arteries and blood from 390 males ages 15 to 34 who died accidentally or violently. Researchers found the most streaks and plaques in men with the highest levels of LDL. And again, they found the fewest streaks and plaques in those with the highest HDL levels.

The researchers said their study "strongly supports the view" that controlling blood cholesterol levels "will retard the progression of atherosclerosis in the young."[6]

So what factors cause high blood cholesterol levels in children? "There are basically two: the genetic makeup and diet," said Dr. Jack Strong, one of the PDAY researchers and the director of the pathology department at Louisiana State University's School of Medicine.

With no way to alter children's genetic makeup, doctors emphasize dietary changes to lower their blood cholesterol. "The most important thing is limiting the saturated fats," Dr. Strong said. Dr. McGill, another PDAY researcher, agrees. "We don't know the mechanism, but the evidence that [saturated fat] does raise LDL is very strong," he said. "There's pretty much of a consensus on that among the scientists studying it."

Kids' High-Fat Diet

American children eat too much fat in general, including too much saturated fat. Children ages 1 to 19 get about 34 percent of their calories from fat.[7] By contrast, health authorities agree that children over age 2 should get no more than 30 percent of their calories from all types of fat. Organizations agreeing on the 30 percent maximum include the American Heart Association, National Academy of Sciences, American Academy of Pediatrics, American Health Foundation, National Cancer Institute, and National Cholesterol Education Program of the National Heart, Lung, and Blood Institute, among others.[8] Many experts encourage diets still lower in fat—provided children get enough calories and nutrients.

How does the 30 percent fat recommendation translate into reality for an average child? Consider an 8-year-old boy who eats 2,000 calories per day. If he gets 34 percent of his calories from

Daily Fat Limits for Kids

*H*ealth experts recommend that everyone over the age of 2 eat a diet that receives no more than 30 percent of its calories from fat. A lower fat intake of closer to 25 percent of calories would be even better, though it might be hard for some children to reach that level. Even more important than limiting total fat is to limit saturated fat. Ten percent of calories should be your child's initial target, but 7 percent would be even better. Getting that low means eating very little meat, cheese, and whole milk.

Age	2–3	4–6	7–10	11–18 females	11–14 males	15–18 males
Average calorie intake	1,300	1,800	2,000	2,200	2,500	3,000
Fat grams (30% of calories	43	60	67	73	83	100
Fat grams (25% of calories)	36	50	56	61	69	83
Saturated fat grams (10% of calories)	14	20	22	24	28	33
Saturated fat grams (7% of calories)	10	14	17	17	19	23

Calorie data taken from Recommended Dietary Allowances, *National Academy of Sciences, 10th ed. (1989).*

the total amount of fat he eats, that translates into 76 grams of fat daily. (Each gram of fat has 9 calories.) If he gets 30 percent or less of his calories from fat, he would consume no more than 67 grams of fat. To meet the guidelines, the boy would have to cut at least 9 grams of fat from his daily diet. A diet getting 25 percent of its calories from fat would contain 56 grams of fat.

To put these numbers in perspective, a typical hot dog has 13 grams of fat, one ounce of potato chips has about 11 grams, a McDonald's Big Mac has 26 grams, and a KFC Original Recipe chicken thigh has 20 grams. Clearly, it shouldn't be too hard for most children to drop 9 or even more grams of fat from their daily diet. Judging from a 1994 Cornell University study, some of the greatest opportunities for cutting back on fat would be for children to drink less whole milk, and eat fewer cookies, cakes, and hot dogs and other luncheon meats.[9]

Most authorities are even more concerned about saturated fat, the type of fat linked to heart disease. Children over age 2 should get less than 10 percent of their calories from saturated fat, according to the experts. American children now eat about one-third more than the recommended amount.[10]

According to the Cornell study, whole milk and cheese are major sources of saturated fat in kids' diets. Switching from whole milk, ice cream, and regular cheese to 1 percent or skim milk, low-fat or fat-free frozen yogurt, and low-fat cheese can help reduce their saturated fat intake while ensuring they still obtain the calcium and other essential nutrients that are abundant in dairy foods. To cut saturated fat from meat, switch from untrimmed meats (or untrimmable meats—like regular hot dogs, hamburgers, and bologna) to trimmed round steak or to hot dogs and luncheon meats that are labeled low-fat. "Lean" meats and ground beef are lower but *not* low in fat. If you search the meat counter, you may be able to find one or two brands of low-fat ground beef, such as Healthy Choice's Extra Lean Ground Beef. Nutritious vegetarian hot dogs and burgers

Babies Need Fat in Their Diets

Every group that advocates reducing children's fat and cholesterol intakes adds an important caveat: Parents should not cut fat and cholesterol in the diets of children under age 2. Infants and 1-year-olds need high levels of fat for proper growth. Mothers' milk gets about 50 percent of its calories from fat.

If parents reduce fat and cholesterol too early, "there is the possibility that there will be problems in terms of maturation of body organs like the liver, spleen, kidneys, and brain, because of the tremendous growth that goes on in the first two years of life," said Dr. Richard Garcia, a pediatrician who co-directs the Cleveland Clinic's pediatric fats clinic.

There have been a few rare cases where well-meaning but misinformed parents dramatically cut their infants' fat and cholesterol consumption. The parents feared that their children would become obese, develop heart disease, or adopt unhealthy eating habits. In the most extreme cases, the lack of calories stunted the infants' growth.* Once the children started eating a regular diet, normal growth resumed.

---

*See, for example, Michael Pugliese et al., "Parental Health Beliefs as a Cause of Nonorganic Failure to Thrive," *Pediatrics*, 80, No. 2 (August 1987), 175.

are increasingly available and tasty. Other major sources of saturated fat in kids' diets include poultry, butter and margarine, cookies, fries, and chips.

In general, the unsaturated fats—monounsaturated and polyunsaturated—do *not* raise blood cholesterol levels. And polyunsaturated fats may even slightly lower cholesterol levels in blood.

One kind of fat deserves special mention: partially hydrogenated vegetable oils, which are found in vegetable shortening, most margarines, and many other processed foods. Oils are hydrogenated to make them harder, such as with stick-type margarines, and more resistant to spoilage. But the hydrogenation process reduces the amount of polyunsaturated fats, raises the amount of saturated fat, and creates *trans* fats. *Trans* fats are monounsaturated, but still raise blood cholesterol levels about as much as saturated fats.[11] Aside from shortening and margarine, *trans* fats are present in baked goods, chips, fried fast foods, and any other foods containing partially hydrogenated vegetable oil.

The fact that most unsaturated fats don't cause heart disease doesn't mean that your children may consume unlimited amounts of them. As we'll discuss shortly, all types of fat are linked to increased cancer risk. And all fats are fattening. A gram of fat has more than twice as many calories as a gram of protein or carbohydrate—and it's easier for the body to convert fatty foods to fat bellies and thighs.[12] The bottom line: Lower your child's intake of *all* types of fat, but especially saturated fat.

One word of caution, though: Don't restrict your child's diet to less than about 25 percent of calories from fat. Children need energy (calories), and a diet very low in fat may stunt a child's growth. The Bogalusa Heart Study found that children whose diets contain less than 30 percent of calories from fat tend to consume low levels of several B vitamins. Dr. Theresa Nicklas and her colleagues who conducted the study said that focusing on low fat intake is not enough. "Equal attention needs to be given to educating the public on the importance of a well-balanced intake . . . ," they said. Children eating low-fat diets ate much less meat but many more sugary candies and soft drinks than those eating high-fat diets.[13] To make up for nutrients like iron and zinc that are found in fatty meat, children need to eat more beans, vegetables, and grains.

Dietary Cholesterol—
The Other Culprit

While saturated and *trans* fats are the prime culprits in raising blood cholesterol, they are not the only ones. Dietary cholesterol—the cholesterol found in foods—also can boost cholesterol levels in blood.

The impact that dietary cholesterol has on blood cholesterol levels varies widely from individual to individual. "There are some people who are highly susceptible to dietary cholesterol, and some who are quite resistant to it," said Dr. McGill of the Southwest Foundation for Biomedical Research. "The mechanism of why some are susceptible and some are resistant is probably genetic, but we don't know which genes yet."

Only foods from animal sources contain cholesterol. Egg yolks are the major source of cholesterol in the average child's diet, but dairy products, meat, and cookies and cakes also provide a significant amount. Many of those foods—particularly fatty dairy and meat products—also have high levels of saturated fat that further raise blood cholesterol. That should make you doubly careful not to include too much of them in your children's diet.

Because dietary cholesterol helps boost blood cholesterol levels, children over the age of 2 should consume no more than about 200 milligrams to 300 milligrams daily.

However, one in three children ages 2 to 18 eats more than 300 milligrams of cholesterol a day.[14] And some children consume astronomical amounts. For example, a study of Cin-

Cholesterol Counts

To put the recommended daily maximum of 200 to 300 milligrams of cholesterol in context, here's the amount of cholesterol in a few foods kids commonly eat.

• A large egg: 213 milligrams

• A cup of whole milk: 33 milligrams
• A Wendy's Double Cheeseburger: 145 milligrams
• A Supreme Personal Pan Pizza from Pizza Hut: 49 milligrams

cinnati schoolchildren found that 10 percent of boys ages 13 to 15 ate 967 milligrams or more of cholesterol daily. Among girls ages 13 to 15, 10 percent ate at least 555 milligrams of cholesterol daily.[15] Although surveys by the federal government show that a disproportionate number of children who consume high levels of cholesterol are poor, and have poorly educated parents, many middle-class kids have high levels.[16]

The single best way to reduce cholesterol is to feed your children fewer egg yolks. Next, switch to fat-free dairy products. And third, replace some of the meat and poultry in their diets with vegetables, whole grains, and beans.

Today, researchers are continuing to explore the link between kids' intake of fat and cholesterol and their risk of heart disease. Yet it's already clear that kids' blood cholesterol levels affect their risk of suffering heart disease later in life. And other than genetics, nothing affects kids' cholesterol levels more than diet. "Everything points toward a balanced diet of natural foods with lots of vegetables and fruits, less meat, and less fat as being the healthiest diet," Dr. McGill said. "That's the kind of diet that parents should get their kids started on. They ought to get started enjoying the healthy foods as children and establish a pattern that persists for life."

The Cholesterol Testing Debate

IN AN IDEAL WORLD, doctors could peer inside children's arteries to detect the early signs of heart disease. Children at high risk—those with lots of large lesions—would get medical treatment. Children at low risk—those with fewer, smaller lesions—would not.

Unfortunately, researchers haven't yet developed a quick, cheap way to look inside the arteries. The next best way to determine children's risk of heart disease is to check cholesterol levels in their blood. However a cholesterol test—a simple blood test—isn't a perfect indicator of a child's risk. While many people who have high cholesterol levels as children also do so as adults, some do not. And some who have normal cholesterol levels as children later have high readings.

The inadequacies of cholesterol tests lie at the heart of a big dispute among doctors: Is it worth testing cholesterol levels in all children?

In 1991, the National Cholesterol Education Program (NCEP) at the National Heart, Lung, and Blood Institute recommended that only certain children get their cholesterol levels checked:

- Those with a parent or grandparent who suffered from cardiovascular disease by age 55 or before.
- Those with a parent whose cholesterol level is 240 milligrams or more. In adults, a reading of 240 or more is cause for great concern.

The panel based its recommendation on studies showing that high cholesterol levels and heart disease often run in families. Children at high risk should get their first test any time after age 2, the panel said. If the first test reveals acceptable levels, the child should be tested again five years later. Under the committee's guidelines, about one-quarter of all children ages 2 to 18 would qualify for testing.

The panel said there is "insufficient scientific and medical evidence to recommend universal screening." Some leading cardiologists and health experts strongly disagree. "You're going to miss about one-half the kids [with high cholesterol levels] by using those guidelines," said Dr. Gerald

Berenson, director of the Bogalusa Heart Study.

Recent studies confirm this opinion. In one, doctors at the Cleveland Clinic examined cholesterol tests done on 6,500 children ages 3 to 18. A total of 375 children had high cholesterol levels. Of them, 48 percent had no family history of early heart disease or high cholesterol. Thus, if doctors had only tested children qualifying under the NCEP guidelines, they would have missed about half the children with high cholesterol. The Cleveland doctors concluded that all children should be tested.* Equally troubling, the studies consistently find that far more children have high cholesterol levels than previously believed.

Will the government guidelines eventually change to call for testing cholesterol in all children? It's possible. In the meantime, you have to decide whether to get your child tested. The evidence linking children's cholesterol levels to their development of arterial lesions is compelling. And kids with high cholesterol are three times more likely to have high levels as adults than kids with normal levels.†

Thus, it makes sense to have your child tested between ages 3 and 5. A normal reading will give you peace of mind—but shouldn't lead you to celebrate with a double-cheeseburger-and-fries dinner. A low-fat diet should be every family's standard. On the other hand, a high reading shouldn't cause alarm (for one thing, a single measurement may not be accurate). Instead, it should prompt you, your child, and your pediatrician or dietitian to work together to achieve a normal level. As you do so, be sure not to communicate to your child that he or she is "sick." Instead, you should say that the whole family is going to be eating a healthier diet. Eating that diet is a big step toward ensuring that both you and your child will live long, healthy lives.

---

*Richard Garcia and Douglas Moodie, "Routine Cholesterol Surveillance in Childhood," *Pediatrics*, 84 (1989), 751.

†Statement by Dr. Ronald Lauer, Press Conference on the *Report of the Expert Panel on Blood Cholesterol Levels in Children and Adolescents* (April 8, 1991), 5.

Dietary Fat and Cancer

L owering your children's intake of fat will lower their risk of heart disease. But it also has another benefit: It may reduce their risk of cancer.

About one-third of all cancer deaths in the United States are related to diet, according to the National Cancer Institute (NCI) and the National Research Council (NRC) of the National Academy of Sciences. That's the same percentage caused by tobacco smoke.[17] Cancer is the nation's second biggest killer, right behind heart disease.

Fat is the dietary substance most strongly linked to cancer, according to the NRC's Committee on Diet, Nutrition, and Cancer. Both population studies and animal experiments "provide convincing evidence that increasing the intake of total fat increases the incidence of cancer at certain sites, particularly the breast and colon," the panel said.

The U.S. Surgeon General's 1988 *Report on Nutrition and Health* agreed. Population studies show "that death rates for cancers of the breast, colon, and prostate are directly proportional to estimated dietary fat intakes," it said.[18]

What influence does a child's fat intake have on her or his cancer risk? No one knows for sure. "Few studies have looked at dietary patterns in children and the impact of these on cancer risk in later life," said Carolyn Clifford, a nutrition expert at the National Cancer Institute.

One of the biggest problems in correlating kids' diets with cancer is cancer's typically long latency period. "We believe it starts maybe 20 or more years before you see the impact," said Regina Ziegler, a researcher who studies diet and cancer at NCI. A thorough study would have to follow thousands of children throughout their entire lifetime. But that's virtually impossible to do, said Dr. Myron Winick, a pediatrician who's professor emeri-

Hot Dogs in the Dog House

In early 1994, a study done at the University of Southern California found high rates of luekemia in children who consumed 12 or more hot dogs a month. That study was very preliminary but indicated the need for additional research. Whether or not its findings are ever confirmed, their high fat and sodium levels already give us enough reasons to cut back on hot dogs in our children's diets.

tus at Columbia University's College of Physicians and Surgeons.

Without such a study, Dr. Winick said, researchers must extrapolate from studies of animals, adults, and entire populations, then add a dose of common sense. "If we put those two together, then I think you could make a case that long-term eating habits will affect the risk of cancer," he said.

The National Cancer Institute agrees. Its dietary recommendation is the same as the one made by other health organizations to lower the risk of heart disease: All people over age 2 should get 30 percent or less of their calories from fat. Other respected organizations make more stringent recommendations, at least for adults. The American Health Foundation notes that animal studies indicate that diets must be no higher than 20 percent fat in order to reduce the risk of cancer. It recommends 25 percent of calories or less as a target. (Traditional Asian diets get closer to 10 percent of calories from fat.)

Most research indicates that fat functions chiefly as a cancer "promoter," rather than as a carcinogen that alters the genetic material in cells. Scientists don't know exactly how fat may promote tumors—and it may vary from breast to colon to prostate cancer. But researchers agree that promoters increase the risk of cancer over a long period of time.[19]

In adults, diets high in fat are most clearly linked to cancer of the colon, which kills 50,000 Americans each year.[20] Studies show that:

- Populations that eat more fat have higher rates of colon cancer.
- Animals fed a cancer-causing chemical get more colon tumors when they're fed a high-fat diet.
- Fatty diets increase the amounts in the stool of bile acids, which can promote cancer.[21]

Recent studies provide evidence that animal fat in particular may be the culprit. The Nurses Health Study, conducted by the Harvard Medical School, studied more than 80,000 women for six years.[22] "The risk of colon cancer was almost double for women who ate the most animal fat compared to those who ate the least," says Harvard's Dr. Meir Stampfer.

Red meat seems largely to blame. The risk of colon cancer was highest for women who ate almost five ounces of red meat per day, and lowest for those who ate no more than two ounces.

A study of male health professionals also found a higher risk of colon cancer in people who eat more animal fat, especially from red meat. Vegetable fat did not appear to promote colon cancer.[23]

Prostate cancer may also be more closely linked to animal fats than to vegetable fats. Harvard researchers analyzed diet questionnaires obtained in 1986 from 47,855 healthy male health professionals.[23] After four years, 126 had developed advanced prostate cancer, the second most deadly cancer (after lung) in American men. The risk of advanced prostate cancer was more than twice as high among men who reported eating the most fat from red meat. Fat from fish, vegetable oils, poultry without the skin, and dairy products other than butter was not linked to a higher risk, although the study did not definitively clear them of blame.

"We need to confirm these results with further studies," cautions Harvard's Dr. Edward Giovannucci. In the meantime, his advice to red-meat-eaters is "The less, the better."

Many more studies have focused on the possible link between diet and breast cancer, which kills 46,000 women a year.[25] To date, the results are mixed, with some researchers finding that women who eat high-fat diets have a greater breast cancer risk. Other researchers have not found such a correlation.

The National Research Council's Committee on Diet and Health examined all the studies on fat and breast cancer. It concluded that "fat intake early in life may have a greater influence on breast cancer risk than intake later in life."[25]

Reducing a child's cancer risk requires lowering his or her total fat intake. While recommendations for preventing heart disease emphasize reducing *saturated* fat, there's no such emphasis with cancer.

Just as with heart disease, researchers will probably never be able to prove conclusively that what kids eat affects their later risk of cancer. Yet for both heart disease and cancer, the evidence strongly suggests that kids' diets influence their risk.

Fortunately, the diets recommended for preventing heart disease and cancer are remarkably similar. "I think we're beginning to deal now with an overall eating pattern that is important in the lowering of risk of a number of different diseases," Dr. Winick said. Such a diet emphasizes eating less fat and cholesterol, eating more fiber-containing whole grains and beans, increasing consumption of fruits and vegetables, and maintaining an ideal body weight. "All of these things are really important not only for cancer, but for heart disease and for the general health of the child," he said.

Eating such a diet will not make your child immune to heart disease and cancer. Other factors besides diet affect the onset and progression of both diseases. Yet with heart disease and cancer ranking as the top two killers of Americans, it clearly makes sense to do everything possible to lower your child's risk.

CHAPTER 2

Sugar and Salt

For many years, sugar was probably the most reviled ingredient in the American diet. Some parents and doctors—and most dentists—cast sugar as the arch nutritional ogre, responsible for causing everything from dental cavities to hyperactivity in children.

More recently, salt—or sodium chloride—has gotten lots of attention. The concern is that children who eat lots of salt are likelier to suffer from high blood pressure as adults.

American children do eat too much sugar and salt, but you may be surprised by what problems they cause (and don't cause). In this chapter, we'll explain how eating too much sugar and salt can be harmful to your children's health. We'll also discuss why it's important to limit your children's sugar and salt intake from an early age.

Happily, if you limit how much fat your children eat, as we described in the previous chapter, you may also reduce their sugar intake. That's because some foods high in fat and cholesterol, such as pies, pastry, chocolate, and ice cream, also contain lots of sugar. And if you reduce the role of processed foods in your children's diets, you'll probably cut their sodium intake.

Sugar

Sugar deserves much of the scorn it has received over the years. It has no nutritional value other than providing calories. The calories from sugar are "empty calories," because sugar itself contains no vitamins, minerals, protein, or fiber.

Too many empty calories in the diet can be a problem for everyone, especially when rates of childhood obesity are soaring. While sugar does provide energy that kids need, each calorie children waste on sugar is one less they can spend eating a nutrient-dense food that will aid proper growth and development. It's important for all of us, children and adults alike, to make each calorie as nutrient-dense as possible to get the maximum benefit from the foods we eat.

Almost everyone craves sugar. "We're born with an innate liking for sweets," said Leann Birch, a professor at the University of Illinois who studies children's food preferences. The genetic preference for a sweet taste may have helped *Homo sapiens* survive in their early days. According to one theory, the preference spurred early humans to eat sweet fruits, which contain lots of nutrients, especially vitamin C.

In the twentieth century, Americans—particularly children—have taken their fondness of sweetness to an extreme. Today, children between ages 1 and 18 get about a quarter of their calories from sugars, including both naturally occurring and refined sugars.[1] On average, Americans eat more than twice as much refined sugar now than they did a hundred years ago. And, despite the rising popularity of artificial sweeteners, consumption of refined sugars also continues to rise.

So what impact does all this sugar have on children's health and their long-term risk of disease? Some authorities contend that except for promoting dental cavities, sugar is basically harmless. That was the conclusion of a Sugars Task Force convened by the U.S. Food and Drug Administration.

That exoneration is not appropriate, especially when so many questions remain about sugar. Sugar may not be the monster that some have claimed it is. Yet it's also not a "safe and high-quality food that plays an important role in a balanced diet," as is claimed by the Sugar Association, an industry group.[2] The truth lies somewhere between those extremes.

Replacing Nutritious Foods

While naturally occurring and refined sugars are chemically identical, there is still an important difference between them: Naturally occurring sugars in fruit and milk are accompanied by valuable vitamins and minerals; fruits also contain fiber and "phytochemicals" that may reduce the risk of cancer. All those nutrients more than make up for the sugar content.

Refined sugar is a different story. Whether it's added at the table, during cooking, or during processing, refined sugar contributes nothing but empty calories. Soft drinks are probably the biggest source of added sugar in the average child's diet. A 12-ounce can of Coke contains about ten teaspoons of added sugar, along with flavorings, water, and caffeine. The Coke gets all of its 144 calories from sugar. They are truly empty calories, since the Coke contributes no nutrients other than calories to the diet.

In the first few years of life, kids get slightly more of their calories from naturally occurring sugars than from added sugars. That's because most kids are still eating lots of fruit and drinking lots of milk and haven't yet discovered soft drinks. But by age 4, added sugars take precedence. By the teen years, on average kids get 14 percent of their calories from added sugars, and one-tenth of teenagers get at least 20 percent of their total calories from added sugar.[3]

Children who eat a lot of sugar can have trouble getting

A Sugar By Any Other Name . . .

When you check a food's ingredient list, sugar can appear in many disguises. Some foods contain several kinds of sugar. Here are some types of sugar you may see:

Corn syrup	High-fructose corn syrup	Maple syrup
Dextrose	Honey	Molasses
Fructose	Lactose	Sucrose
Glucose	Maltose	

enough nutrients. That's because they must get 100 percent of their nutrients from just 80 or 85 percent of their food. That's hard to do.

Patricia Guenther, a nutritionist at the U.S. Department of Agriculture, has found that soft drinks "have the greatest impact on the adequacy of calcium intake." Both boys and girls who consumed one or more soft drinks a day tended to consume about one-fifth less calcium than children who did not drink soft drinks. Guenther noted that many children drink soft drinks with meals and figured "that teenagers may be substituting soft drinks for milk at meals."[4]

This is a special problem, because milk is one of the best sources of calcium, and it is crucial that children consume enough in order to build up their bones. If they don't, they will be likelier to develop osteoporosis (brittle-bone disease) later in life. (Grammar-school kids should consume at least two glasses of skim or 1 percent milk or yogurt a day, and older children at least three; children can also get significant amounts of calcium from other dairy products; fortified bread, cereal, and 100 percent juice; sardines; kale; tofu; and other foods, as well as calcium supplements.)

If you're trying to get at least five servings a day of fresh fruits

Sugar Levels in Common Foods

Food	Serving Size	Sugar (grams)
Beverages		
Minute Maid Orange soda	12 oz	48
Coca-Cola Classic, Pepsi	12 oz	41
McDonald's chocolate shake	10 oz	38
Hawaiian Punch Double C	1 cup	28
Minute Maid Lemonade	1 cup	26
chocolate milk—2 percent fat	1 cup	15
Sauces, Spreads, and Condiments		
Hungry Jack, Regular Syrup	¼ cup	28
Mott's Original Apple Sauce (individual containers)	½ cup	18
Prego Traditional Spaghetti Sauce	½ cup	14
Pastries, Desserts, and Yogurt		
Dannon Raspberry Yogurt (lowfat)	1 cup	43
Hostess Sno Balls	1 pkg	35
Yoplait Trix	¾ cup	25
Hostess Twinkies	1 pkg	25
Good Humor Breyers Ice Cream Sandwich	1	22
Good Humor Breyers Fudgsicle	1	20
Swiss Miss Vanilla Pudding Snack	½ cup	19
Good Humor Breyers Garfield Bar	1	17
Oreos	3 cookies	13
Krispy Kreme Glazed Doughnuts	1 (38 g)	11

Quaker Chewy Granola Bars	1 bar (28 g)	8–9
Teddy Grahams, cinnamon or chocolate	24 (1 oz)	8–9

Cereals

Instant Oatmeal—Cinnamon & Spice or Raisins & Spice	1 packet	15
Apple Jacks	1 oz (1 cup)	14
Froot Loops	1 oz (1 cup)	13
Kellogg's Frosted Flakes	1 oz (¾ cup)	13
Cap'n Crunch	1 oz (¾ cup)	12
Lucky Charms	1 oz (1 cup)	12
Life	1 oz (⅔ cup)	5
Ralston Corn Chex	1 oz (1¼ cup)	3
Wheaties	1 oz (1 cup)	3
Kellogg's Corn Flakes	1 oz (1 cup)	2
Cheerios	1 oz (1¼ cup)	1

Candies

3 Musketeers	2.1 oz bar	40
Reese's Pieces	2.7oz	40
M & M's plain	1 bag (1.7 oz)	31
Snickers	1 bar (2.1 oz)	29
Twizzlers Strawberry Twists	2.5 oz pkg	26
Hershey's Chocolate Bar	1.55 oz bar	22
Chunky	1.4 oz	20
Reese's Peanut Butter Cups	1.6 oz pkg	19
Kit-Kat	1 pkg	18

Sources: manufacturers; Center for Science in the Public Interest

and vegetables into your child's diet, make sure that he or she does not fill up on sugary doodads. At breakfast, provide a low-sugar cereal, like shredded wheat, Wheaties or Cheerios, with banana slices instead of a sugary cereal. Offer an orange or apple at snack time rather than a candy bar. And for dessert serve a vitamin-packed slice of watermelon instead of a piece of cake.

Of course, some kids don't *replace* the nutritious foods in their diet with sugar-laden goodies. Instead, they pile the sugary foods *on top* of their normal diet. That promotes obesity, a major problem for millions of children.

Sugar and Tooth Decay

"Sugars are the most important dietary factors in the causation of dental caries," said *The 1988 Surgeon General's Report on Nutrition and Health*. Newly erupting teeth in children are especially at risk. The report recommended that people who are particularly vulnerable to cavities, especially children, eat fewer sugary foods. Interestingly, the critical issue isn't how much sugar a child eats. "Rather than talking about the amount of sugar or even the frequency of use of sugar, really the major concept is how much time are the child's teeth exposed to a food source," said Carole Palmer, who teaches nutrition and preventive dentistry at the Tufts University School of Dental Medicine.

Consider two children, each given a candy bar containing five teaspoons of sugar. The first child gobbles down the whole bar at one sitting. The second child carefully breaks it into five pieces and eats a piece every few hours during the day. Which child has a greater risk of getting cavities? The answer is the second child, even though the two children ate the same amount of sugar. That's because the second child's teeth were in contact with sugar for a much longer period.

The form in which a child eats sugar also affects the level of risk. For example, crackers and sugary cereals are more likely than soda pop to cause cavities. The reason is that sticky foods adhere to teeth, while the soda washes off quickly. Of course, someone who slowly sucks on several bottles of soda pop in a day will keep his or her teeth bathed in sugar water for a long time. Surprisingly, caramels and jelly beans don't stay on teeth as long as mixtures of starch and sugar, like breakfast cereals.[5]

Naturally occurring sugars have just as much potential to cause cavities as the sugar in a cereal. However, the sugars in, say, fruit are diluted and don't stick to teeth, which lessens their threat. Nonetheless, parents should not put an infant to bed with a bottle of fruit juice (or milk, for that matter) because of the risk of cavities.

The good news about tooth decay is that, despite their virtual addiction to sugar, American children have many fewer cavities today than ever before. According to the National Institute of Dental Research (NIDR), in the late 1980s children had 36 percent fewer cavities than did children at the beginning of the decade. That dramatic decline followed a similar drop during the 1970s. "What we're seeing is the beginning of the end for a disease that has plagued mankind throughout history," said Dr. Harald Löe, NIDR's director.[6]

What's causing the drop in children's cavities? According to Palmer, the primary reason is the effectiveness of fluoridation, which provides tooth-strengthening fluoride in drinking water. Fluoride-containing toothpaste also plays a role. Still, children should cut back on sugary snacks and regularly brush their teeth after each meal.

Sugar and Behavioral Problems

One major concern of many parents is whether sugar causes behavioral problems in children. The evidence on that issue remains mixed. Most studies have not found that sugar affects behavior, and *The Surgeon General's Report on Nutrition and Health* said the evidence linking sugar (as well as caffeine and certain food additives) to behavioral problems is "weak and contradictory." As with food additives (see Chapter 4), sugar does not have as widespread or severe effects as many parents believe. However, it does affect some children—especially younger ones.

For examples of the mixed evidence linking sugar and behavior, consider the results of several studies:

- A study of hyperactive children found that sugar decreased the kids' attention span.[7] Remarkably, that study was sponsored by the sugar industry.
- A study of non-hyperactive children found that sugar caused more inappropriate behavior while the kids were playing.[8]
- Dr. Judith Rapoport and her colleagues at the National Institute of Mental Health found that sugar actually quieted down some grade-school children who were thought by their parents to be sensitive to sugar. However, sugar did cause 3 out of 21 children in their study to be more active.[9]
- The most recent study, done at Vanderbilt University, did not find any effect on 26 6- to 10-year-olds whose parents thought they were sensitive to sugar.[10]

The studies indicate that sugar does not dramatically affect most kids and is not a common cause of hyperactivity. But it does appear to have modest effects on some children.

If you think your child is sensitive to sugar, you can try a little test. C. Keith Conners, professor of medical psychology at Duke University Medical Center, suggests giving your child sugar, both with and without protein-rich foods like milk, meat, or cheese. Each time, watch how your child reacts. Observation "is really the only sensible approach" to determining whether a child reacts to sugar, Conners said. "There is no test of a physiological nature. It really requires empirical observation." (It's best to try the test several times to minimize the effect of non-food influences on your child's behavior.)

Another test involves eliminating as much honey and sugar—including sucrose, corn syrup, corn sugar, glucose, dextrose, and high-fructose corn syrup—as you can from your child's diet and then watching for behavior changes. But remember that soft drinks, candy, and many other sugary foods also contain numerous additives that might be responsible for any behavior changes. (See page 70 for a description of a test you can do to determine if your child is sensitive to foods or ingredients.)

Sodium

American children eat far more salt than they need. Although little research has been done with children, there's strong evidence that all this salt—or sodium chloride—is boosting their chances of developing high blood pressure as adults. High blood pressure, or hypertension, is a major risk factor for strokes and heart disease. Strokes killed 145,000 Americans in 1990, while coronary heart disease killed 489,000 more.[11] Obesity is the biggest cause of high blood pressure, but for many people salt is also a significant factor.

The body needs just a small amount of sodium. A 1-year-old child needs only 225 milligrams of sodium daily. That's less than is in a couple of slices of bread or a cup of most breakfast cereals. The amount needed slowly rises with age, but by age 18 kids still need just 500 milligrams daily.[12] By contrast, the Bogalusa Heart Study found that by age 2, the average child ate

Sodium's Stage Names

Most of the sodium in our diet comes from the added salt and a variety of additives and seasonings in processed foods. Some of the most common ingredients that provide sodium include:

Salt	Sodium benzoate
Baking powder	Sodium caseinate
Baking soda	Sodium citrate
Celery salt	Sodium erythorbate
Garlic salt	Sodium nitrate
Monosodium glutamate (MSG)	Sodium phosphate
Onion salt	Sodium propionate
Seasoned salt	Sodium saccharin
Sodium ascorbate	Sodium tripolyphosphate

2,670 milligrams of sodium daily, and sodium intake rose steadily with age. By age 17, the average child ate 3,670 milligrams of sodium daily.[13] Thus, children typically eat about five to ten times more sodium than they need.[14]

The National Research Council of the National Academy of Sciences recommends that everyone over age 2 eat no more than 2,400 milligrams of sodium daily. Eating just 1,800 milligrams daily would be even better, the council says. That's equivalent to about one teaspoon of salt. But if you think your child's diet is low in sodium because he or she rarely uses a salt-shaker, think again: The vast majority of the sodium Americans consume comes from the salt and other sodium-containing chemicals found in processed foods.

Americans get about three-quarters of their sodium from processed foods.[15] Lots of processed foods aimed at kids have extremely high sodium levels, but you can't always tell the sodium content from the taste. For example, you'd think that potato chips and french fries would be high in sodium because they taste salty. However, one ounce of potato chips (about 14 chips) has only about 135 milligrams, and a large pack of McDonald's french fries has 200 milligrams. By contrast, an average hot dog has 500 milligrams, a Bacon Double Cheeseburger Deluxe at Burger King has 748 milligrams, and a Roast Chicken Club Sandwich at Arby's has 1,423 milligrams. When salt is just sprinkled on the outside of a food, as with potato chips and french fries, there might not be as much there as your taste buds perceive. But when it's mixed throughout the food, such as in a bun or soup, huge amounts may be present.

Some of the evidence that kids should reduce their salt intake comes from the Bogalusa Heart Study in Louisiana. Dr. Gerald Berenson, director of the study, said he and his colleagues found that hypertension begins in childhood and that "diet is a major factor" in its onset. Children whose blood pressure ranks high compared to their peers are likely to have high blood pressure as adults, too.

The best evidence that sodium is important in youth's high blood pressure comes from a study done by Dr. Alan Sinaiko and his colleagues at the University of Minnesota Medical School. The researchers identified 210 boys and girls in the fifth to eighth grades who had high blood pressure. Some of the children were put on a low-sodium diet; others were given a potassium supplement or a placebo. Over the three-year study, the systolic (the second of the two numbers) blood pressure of girls who restricted their sodium to about 1,500 milligrams a day decreased an average of 1.5 millimeters. According to the researchers, that modest reduction in blood pressure could have a significant effect on health. The blood pressure of the girls taking the placebo increased by about 4 millimeters.

The boys, however, did not fare so well. They refused to stick to a low-sodium diet and their blood pressure increased.

Sodium Levels in Common Foods

Food	Serving Size	Sodium (milligrams)
Dairy		
cottage cheese	½ cup	445
American cheese	1 oz	335
cheddar cheese	1 oz	185
chocolate milk—2 percent fat	1 cup	150
milk	1 cup	120
Breads, Cereals, and Snacks		
pretzels	1 oz	515
Kellogg's Corn Flakes	1 oz (1¼ cup)	350
bread	2 slices	300
Cheerios	1 oz (1¼ cup)	290
potato chips	15	135
Meats		
Oscar Mayer Healthy Favorites Bologna	2 oz	655
salami, beef	2 oz	655
hot dog, Oscar Mayer Beef Frank	1 (1.6 oz)	450
bacon, cooked	3 medium pieces	303
tuna, light, canned in water, drained	2 oz	190
Fruits and Vegetables		
Campbell's Light 'N Tangy V8 Vegetable Juice	1 cup	320

peas, frozen	½ cup	70
carrot	1 medium	25
corn	½ cup	15
apple, banana, orange, or peach	1 medium	0

Sauces and Spreads

Prego Meat Flavored Spaghetti Sauce	½ cup	660
Healthy Choice Chunky Spaghetti Sauce	½ cup	350
peanut butter	2 Tbsp.	260
ketchup	1 Tbsp.	155
mayonnaise	1 Tbsp.	80

Prepared Foods

Domino's Pepperoni Pizza	2 slices, 12" regular crust	1,150
Chef Boyardee Spaghetti 'n Meatballs in Tomato Sauce	7.5 oz (½ can)	1,140
Campbell's Chicken Noodle Soup	1 cup	870
McDonald's Cheeseburger	1	730
Kraft Macaroni and Cheese	1 cup	710
McDonald's Egg McMuffin	1	710
Taco Bell Chicken Soft Taco	1	615
Campbell's Healthy Request Chicken Noodle Soup	1 cup	470
McDonalds French Fries	medium	150

Sources: manufacturers; *Bowes and Church's Food Values of Portions Commonly Used*, Jean A. T. Pennington, New York: HarperPerennial, 1989; *Nutrition Action Healthletter*

According to Dr. Sinaiko, it was the high-salt food the boys ate outside the home "that really did them in."

In addition to high blood pressure, new research is showing that lifelong diets high in sodium increase the risk of osteoporosis. When the body excretes the excess sodium, a little calcium goes out with it. Eating an extra teaspoon of salt (about 2,000 milligrams of sodium) each day causes the body to excrete enough calcium to dissolve about 1 percent of bone annually. Over a decade, that's 10 percent of a person's skeleton.[16]

If that's not enough reason to keep sodium levels down, recent research has also implicated high-sodium diets in stomach cancer. While the rate of stomach cancer among Americans has declined precipitously since the 1930s, this disease still kills 25,000 people a year. People with stomach cancer tend to have consumed larger amounts of salt than the general population. The salt irritates the stomach lining, causing cells to reproduce more rapidly. Salt may also make cancer-causing chemicals more potent.[17]

In the face of all this, Dr. Jeffrey Cutler, who studies cardiovascular disease prevention at the National Heart, Lung, and Blood Institute and co-authored the hypertension chapter in *The Surgeon General's Report on Nutrition and Health,* strongly supports limiting the amount of salt that kids eat. "Tastes are acquired early," he said. "Once acquired they can be changed, but changing them is harder than not acquiring them in the first place. If you're used to eating food relatively low in salt, it won't take much added salt to make certain foods taste better. . . . But the more you're used to, the more it takes to get that pleasurable taste. To me, that all points in the direction of an early approach."

Rose Stamler, professor of epidemiology at the Northwestern Medical School in Chicago, estimates that if Americans cut their sodium intake in half—from two teaspoons of salt a day to one—the death rate from heart disease would drop by 5 percent and from hypertension by 9 percent.

Some people figure they can eat lots of salt until a doctor says they're hypertensive, at which point they can cut back. That's a nice theory, but it doesn't always work in practice. "Once induced by a high sodium intake, blood pressure is not necessarily corrected by resumption of a moderately low intake," said the National Research Council.[18]

That argues for moderating salt intake starting in childhood. Even if your children have already learned to love salt, you can help them unlearn it. People who reduce their salt intake for several months usually find that their taste buds end up preferring less salt. As a bonus, those people can actually taste the natural flavors of food again, too.

To cut your kids' salt intake, feed them natural rather than processed foods whenever possible. Grains, fruits, vegetables, and most other natural foods have very little sodium. Milk has slightly more, about 120 milligrams per glass. But that's dwarfed by the 500 milligrams to 1,000 milligrams found in canned soup, fast-food hamburgers, and many other processed foods. So check labels carefully for sodium content. You can also add less salt during cooking and replace the saltshaker at the table with an herb shaker.

Hypertension is a disease that's largely preventable. Wouldn't it be nice if our children's generation enjoyed much lower rates of hypertension than their parents?

CHAPTER 3

The Obesity Epidemic

A merica is raising a generation of butterballs. That would be one thing if we were talking about turkeys, but we're not. We're talking about children. Childhood obesity is zooming out of control. At least one child in five is obese, according to Dr. William Dietz, a pediatrician at the Tufts University School of Medicine who specializes in childhood nutrition. Many researchers consider people obese if they're more than 20 percent over the ideal weight for their sex, height, and age. People more than 40 percent over their ideal weight are considered extremely obese.

From 1963 to 1980, obesity among 6- to 11-year-olds grew 54 percent, according to research by Dr. Dietz and his colleagues. Extreme obesity rose in this age group by an astounding 98 percent. Among 12- to 17-year olds, obesity rose 39 percent, and extreme obesity grew 64 percent.[1]

The Bogalusa Heart Study, which examined thousands of children in an effort to determine the links between diet and early signs of heart disease, found a similar increase in childhood obesity. In the 1973–74 school year, about one out of seven 5- to 14-year-old children was overweight. Eleven years later, about one in four children in the same age range was overweight—a 62-percent increase.[2] And researchers who studied children of military personnel discovered almost a doubling of grossly obese children between 1978 and 1986–1990.[3]

As this book went to press, the government was reviewing the most current—and depressing—national statistics on changes in childhood obesity rates between about 1980 and 1990. Preliminary figures appeared to corroborate the earlier studies. Rates of severe obesity among 6- and 11-year-olds appeared to have increased sharply. Among 12- to 17-year-olds, rates may have actually doubled. As many as one out of six African-American girls and young Mexican-American boys and girls is obese.

Two major factors determine whether a child becomes obese: genetics and lifestyle. A child's genes can make him or her susceptible to obesity. However, many children who have "fatness" genes may not actually become obese unless a lack of exercise or poor diet triggers their genetic vulnerability.

What's causing the increase in childhood obesity? Dr. Dietz blames television viewing for one-fourth of the jump. The average child between ages 2 and 5 watches nearly 28 hours of television weekly, according to Nielsen Media Research. The average 6- to 11-year-old watches almost 24 hours, and teens watch 21 to 22 hours.[4] Those figures don't include the additional time spent watching movies on the VCR or playing video games. Thus, the average child likely spends 25 to 30 hours plunked in front of the tube each week, and millions of children spend many more. Years ago, those hours might have been spent exercising and burning off calories.

According to a study by Dr. Dietz and a colleague, among 12- to 17-year-olds the prevalence of obesity rose with each additional hour spent watching TV.[5] Children's metabolic rates may decline while they watch TV, and many kids snack while watching. Both may account for television's connection to obesity.[6]

It's uncertain what other factors have contributed to the rise in childhood obesity, Dr. Dietz said. He suggested, though, that fatty diets and sedentary lifestyles could be important. Some other factors that may play a part include:

- Fast-food restaurants and vending machines are far more prevalent than they used to be. Most fast foods and vended foods are high in calories, fat, or sugar.
- Many kids eat fewer nutritious meals at home with their families. Instead, they snack on soft drinks, chips, candy bars, and fast foods.
- Many kids return to an empty house after school and eat junk food while they watch television.
- Stressed-out family life undermines healthy eating habits.

Obese children face an increased risk of serious health problems, as well as traumatic social and psychological difficulties, in both childhood and adulthood. In childhood, obesity can cause high blood pressure, high blood cholesterol, abnormal glucose tolerance, and—if it's extreme—orthopedic problems such as trouble with walking.[7] Some of these medical problems, such as high cholesterol and high blood pressure, boost the risk of heart disease. Since arteries start clogging in childhood, it's best to get obesity under control at an early age.

Childhood obesity also may raise the risk of cancer later in life, particularly colon and breast cancers, according to David Kritchevsky, a researcher who studies nutrition and degenerative diseases at the Wistar Institute in Philadelphia.

Obesity also raises the risk of adult-onset (Type-II) diabetes. About one in four obese adults is diabetic. Diabetes can cause blindness, kidney failure, nerve damage in the feet and legs, and clogged arteries.

One recent study compared overweight and lean adolescents by examining their health 55 years later. The researchers found that people who were overweight as kids—regardless of their weight as adults—tended to die earlier. Overweight boys had a greater tendency to develop coronary heart disease, gout, and cancer of the colon and rectum. Overweight girls tended to develop both coronary heart disease and arthritis.[8]

Aside from medical problems, obese children also can suffer a range of psychological and social difficulties. Just think back to grade school. Remember how the kids tormented and shunned their overweight peers? Taunts and snubs undermine an impressionable child's self-esteem, as well as his or her ability to build successful relationships.

Dr. Leonard Taitz, author of *The Obese Child*, has written that " . . . being different or merely at the extreme of the norm may exact a savage penalty. . . . Some [fat children] are merely teased, others are bullied unmercifully, and some are virtually ostracized."[9]

Perhaps the biggest reason to avoid excess weight gain during childhood is that obese children often become obese adults. Both the age at which obesity begins and the degree of obesity influence whether it continues into adulthood. The older and heavier the obese child is, the greater chance he or she has of being an obese adult.

According to several studies, the older the child, the greater the risk that obesity will continue into adulthood, said Dr. Leonard Epstein, a leading specialist in childhood obesity and a psychiatry professor at the University of Pittsburgh School of Medicine. He said the studies show that:

- 41 percent of obese 7-year-olds become obese adults.
- 70 percent of obese 10- to 13-year-olds become obese adults.[10]

The pattern continues through adolescence. More than 80 percent of obese adolescents remain obese as adults, according to the National Research Council.[11]

The severity of the obesity also governs whether it continues. The National Research Council reports that among 7-year-olds:

- For those 30 percent to 45 percent over their ideal weight, just under half will be obese in adulthood.
- Among those 57 percent to 65 percent above ideal weight, about four in five will retain the extra weight in adulthood.
- Of those whose weight is 65 percent or more above the ideal, virtually all will be obese adults.[12]

Children at the greatest risk of becoming obese are those whose parents and siblings are overweight. Studies of identical twins indicate that genes are two to three times more important than environmental factors in determining their body weights later in life.[13] In some cases, though, obesity runs in families because children copy the lifestyles of parents who eat poorly and don't exercise.

If both parents are overweight, their child has an 80-percent chance of being heavy, according to the National Research Council. If neither parent is overweight, however, their child has less than a 10-percent chance of being heavy.[14]

Dr. Epstein said many parents worry unnecessarily about a child who gets a little pudgy. "If both parents are thin and three other kids in the family are all thin and one child is a bit heavy, the odds are pretty good that that child's going to outgrow it," he said. "But the odds are not good the child's going to outgrow it if both parents are heavy and the oldest sibling is heavy."

Eating Disorders

In 1990, 44 percent of girls and 15 percent of boys in high school were trying to lose weight.[15] While many Americans—including children—do need to lose weight, some adolescents and young adults go too far. They develop anorexia nervosa or bulimia, eating disorders that can have deadly results.

Anorexia and bulimia are psychiatric ailments that have physical symptoms. They primarily strike teenage girls and young women, particularly white women from middle- and upper-income families. Both problems usually start with a period of dieting, and researchers believe both may be related to our society's preoccupation with thinness.[16]

Anorexia is the rarer of the two disorders. It occurs in less than 1 percent of females between ages 13 and 20.[17] Anorexics have an unusual fear of becoming fat, so they severely limit how much food they eat. They keep limiting their food intake even after they become emaciated, because they still think of themselves as fat. Self-starvation can cause osteoporosis, as well as fatal heart disease.

Many anorexics have rigid personalities and are concerned with perfectionism, according to *The 1988 Surgeon General's Report on Nutrition and Health.* "Individuals are usually preoccupied with food, thinking about it much of the time, preparing meals for others, and often engaging in bizarre eating rituals," the report said. "Many anorexics engage in very extensive physical exercise. The disorder is also associated with a pervasive sense of personal ineffectiveness."

Anorexics usually come from intact families, and their parents commonly consider them model children. Relatively minor events in adolescence may trigger anorexia. Some researchers believe that psychological trauma or domineering mothers may underlie the disease, according to the Surgeon General's report.

Bulimia is more common. Although estimates vary on its prevalence, surveys in Chicago[18] and Louisiana[19] have found that between 4 percent and 5 percent of high school girls are bulimic. While girls in junior high school can become bulimic, the disorder is more common among those in their late teens and early twenties.

Bulimics usually suffer from depression and are more concerned than normal with their body shape and weight. They repeatedly go on eating binges. In the most extreme cases, bulimics follow the binges with self-induced vomiting or use laxatives or diuretics to "get rid of" the food. As a result, bulimics may suffer loss of dental enamel, dry mouth, problems in pregnancy, and gastrointestinal problems.

Anorexics and bulimics need professional help. Sufferers usually claim they don't have a problem and resist going to the doctor. That means parents must insist on treatment. Doctors or other therapists use a variety of approaches to try to help patients, and a growing number are using family therapy as part of their treatment. Unfortunately, there is no tried and true method for treating either anorexia or bulimia. In many cases, kids just seem to outgrow it.

The Bottom Line on the Waistline

Treading the line between being too fat and too thin can be tough for a child. Growing kids need to eat lots of food, but sometimes their growth rate slows down or spurts ahead. This can cause the child to become either a bit pudgy or a little too thin. As long as the weight imbalance is temporary, there's nothing to worry about. If the weight problem continues, though, the child may need help. Failing to maintain an ideal weight can lead to a wide range of health problems, some of which begin in childhood.

How do you lower your children's risk of developing weight problems or eating disorders? First, feed them the diet we recommend in Chapter 10. That diet emphasizes eating more whole-grain breads and cereals, fruits, vegetables, and other fiber-rich natural foods and eating less fat, cholesterol, sugar, sodium, and processed foods.

But be careful not to overdo it. A healthy diet should be a natural part of a child's life, not a rigid set of restrictions that interfere with his or her self-esteem, social skills, and happiness. Ultra-strict rules may well spur kids to rebel by eating unhealthful foods every chance they get. And kids often grow up hating the foods their parents force them to eat. The presence of junk foods should never be a reason to keep kids from attending or enjoying birthday parties or other celebrations.

Second, turn off the TV and play with your kids or send them outside to get some exercise. Kids involved in hobbies, games, and chores will be too engaged to eat out of boredom.

And last, set a good example. Kids' biggest influence is their parents. If you're a snacking couch potato, you have every reason to expect your children will be the same.

Those three actions don't provide sure-fire protection against obesity and eating problems. However, they greatly reduce the chance your children will join the millions of American kids who are obese or suffer from eating disorders.

CHAPTER 4

Bacteria, Additives, and Pesticides

I f you're like most Americans, you were taught at an early age that the government protects you from a wide range of hazards, including poisons in your food. Top government officials routinely proclaim that the United States has the safest food in the world. It's very comforting to think that an army of white-coated government scientists and inspectors is making sure the food you and your children eat is totally safe.

Unfortunately, that rosy view doesn't quite jibe with reality. The truth is that the government has not done nearly as good a job as it should have of ensuring that the nation's food is safe. It has particularly failed to ensure that the food supply is safe for children.

Bacteria, food additives, and pesticides pose risks ranging from food poisoning to allergic reactions to cancer. Children may be at greatest risk because their immune systems may not be well developed, they consume a large quantity of food relative to their weight, and they will be consuming additives and pesticides for the next 70 or more years. In this chapter, we'll discuss the risks and how you and your children can avoid them wherever possible.

Before diving into the details, let us state at the outset that while there's reason to be concerned about food safety, there's no need to panic. If you are vigilant, it's possible to avoid dangerous bacteria, and, with a few exceptions, even the most problematical additives and pesticides pose risks that are very small to a given individual. However, when that risk is multiplied by millions of consumers, the risks to the general population are significant.

Bacteria

In early 1993 Americans had a grim reminder of the age-old problem of food poisoning. Four children on the West Coast died and hundreds more became ill after eating undercooked fast-food hamburgers at Jack in the Box restaurants. The burgers were tainted with E. coli O157:H7 bacteria. In the 1980s and early 1990s other problems also hit the headlines:

- Six hundred people got salmonella food poisoning after eating at a Taco Bell restaurant in Syracuse, New York.
- Contaminated pasteurized milk from a Chicago dairy caused tens of thousands of cases of salmonella poisoning, including several deaths.
- Mexican-style soft cheese contaminated with listeria killed 47 people in Southern California.
- At least one out of three chickens is contaminated with salmonella or campylobacter.
- Eggs contaminated with salmonella cause thousands of cases of food poisoning.

Food poisoning kills an estimated 9,000 Americans each year.[1] Young children, the elderly, and people with compromised immune systems (people who have AIDS or cancer) are the most susceptible to food poisoning.[2] Food-safety experts generally agree that germs in food pose a much greater health problem than additives, pesticides, or other pollutants.

Food poisoning has become more common in the last several decades, and the germs have been getting hardier. Some bacteria have developed resistance to antibiotics because of the heavy use of antibiotics on farms and by doctors. That's a problem, because it can be difficult for a doctor treating someone infected with antibiotic-resistant bacteria to find an antibiotic that works.

Animal products are the major culprits in food poisoning. Ideally, the government and industry would do a better job of ensuring that red meat, poultry, eggs, and seafood were free of dangerous bacteria. Fishing and the harvesting of shellfish should be barred from contaminated waters, farmers should not send any infected livestock to market, slaughterhouses need to be cleaned up, and temperatures need to be controlled all the way from the fishing boat or packinghouse to the grocer's display case. But no matter how vigorous the government is, we will always have to contend with a certain level of bacteria in our food. That means it is up to you, the consumer, to serve as the final defense against food poisoning.

To minimize the chances of anyone in your family being poisoned by what's on their plates, you need to be careful at the grocery store and in the kitchen. The underlying principles are that most bacteria cannot grow in the cold, they flourish at room or body temperature, and they are killed by high heat. To protect your family:

- Make sure that the food you buy is fresh. Check the "use by" or "sell by" dates on dairy products and other perishables, and be sure that eggs are refrigerated and not cracked. Do not buy "raw" (unpasteurized) dairy products.
- Don't feed honey to babies under one year, because of a risk of botulism.

- Store perishables properly and promptly. Your refrigerator should be 40 degrees or colder and your freezer 0 degrees or colder. Fish can be kept in the refrigerator for one day, hamburger meat and poultry for a day or two, steaks for three to five days. If you won't be cooking a food for a longer period, store it in your freezer. Don't leave raw foods out of the refrigerator for more than a couple of hours. Discard shellfish that died in storage and fish (or any food) that smells rotten.
- Thaw frozen foods in the refrigerator or microwave oven rather than at room temperature.
- Wash produce carefully. It is occasionally contaminated with disease-causing bacteria and commonly contaminated with pesticide residues. Discard moldy cottage cheese, individual cheese slices, yogurt, nuts, flour, rice, bread, cake, and dried beans and peas. You can cut away moldy spots on hard cheese, salami, and firm fruits and vegetables; cut out about an inch beyond the mold.
- Handle food carefully when you are preparing to cook it. Assume that meat, poultry, and fish are contaminated; wash in hot, soapy water anything—your hands, cutting board, knives, etc.—that touched those raw foods before you touch any other food, object, or person.
- Cook meat, fish, poultry, and eggs thoroughly. The inside should be completely cooked. Be especially careful with microwave ovens, which can cook foods unevenly. Do not serve soft-boiled eggs, rare steak, or undercooked chicken or fish. Raw shellfish probably poses the greatest risk of any food. At a restaurant, if a food is not thoroughly cooked, return it.
- Put leftovers in the refrigerator right after you eat. Discard leftovers that were at room temperature for more than two hours (one hour if the temperature is over 90 degrees).

Additives

As a treat, parents across America plunk the following concoction into their children's lunch boxes:

> Sugar, water, enriched flour (niacin [a B vitamin], iron [ferrous sulfate], thiamin mononitrate [B_1], riboflavin [B_2]), corn syrup, partially hydrogenated vegetable and/or animal shortening (contains one or more of: canola oil, corn oil, cottonseed oil, soybean oil, beef fat), cocoa, skim milk; contains 2 percent or less of: modified food starch, whey, leavening (may contain: baking soda, monocalcium phosphate, sodium acid pyrophosphate), salt, calcium sulfate, starch, mono- and diglycerides, cellulose gum, lecithin, polysorbate 60, agar, gelatin, natural and artificial flavor, sodium phosphate, sodium stearoyl lactylate, locust bean gum, chocolate, sodium caseinate; sorbic acid (to retard spoilage).

That's a Hostess cupcake with creamy filling, in case you didn't recognize it.

When they get home from school, some kids eat the following for a snack:

> Corn sugar, sugar, gelatin, fruit-juice concentrates (contains pineapple, orange, apple, grape, and watermelon), citric acid, natural and artificial flavorings, sodium citrate, mineral oil, carnauba wax, artificial coloring (includes Yellow 5, Red 40, Yellow 6, and Blue 1), and hydrogenated soybean oil.

That's Tropical Amazin' Fruit Gummy Bears, made by Hershey Foods.

Some parents take their kids to Wendy's for dinner, where the kids eat a hamburger patty placed in:

> Flour, water, high-fructose corn syrup, lard, buttermilk solids, yeast, vital wheat gluten, salt, calcium sulfate,

sodium stearoyl lactylate, calcium stearoyl-2 lactylate, turmeric, paprika, whey solids, sodium caseinate, monocalcium phosphate, niacin, ferrous sulfate, thiamin hydrochloride, riboflavin, potassium bromate, azodicarbonamide.

That's a Wendy's hamburger bun.

After about the tenth item in those ingredient lists, it's easy to feel lost. Just what the heck is sodium stearoyl lactylate? Or sulfiting agents? Or carnauba wax? And who can pronounce "azodicarbonamide," let alone figure out what it is and whether it's safe?

All those chemicals are food additives. Manufacturers intentionally add nearly 3,000 chemicals to our food during processing. Another 12,000 "indirect additives," such as chemicals used on manufacturing equipment and in food packaging, also can end up in food.[3]

Additives play a variety of roles in food. They can adjust the flavor, change the color, increase the nutrients, stabilize the texture, and preserve the freshness. The average American eats about five pounds of food additives annually, not counting the two most common additives, sugar and salt.

Contrary to the scary articles you might have read, most food additives are safe. In addition, some additives even provide clear benefits. For example, the calcium propionate preservative in baked goods adds calcium to the diet. And if it's convenience that you want, convenience foods would be in the Stone Age were it not for emulsifiers, which keep oil and water from separating.

Yet while most food additives pose no risk, others clearly do. Some have been discovered to cause cancer or other health problems in experimental animals, and we have to presume that they would cause the same problems in humans. In a few cases, additives have caused fatal toxic reactions in people. History is replete with instances where, on the basis of studies indicating risks, the Food and Drug Administration (FDA) banned

Public Pressure Gets Results

Public pressure from parents, scientists, legislators, and consumer advocates has sometimes forced companies to remove potentially harmful additives from children's foods. For example, for years baby-food companies added monosodium glutamate, or MSG, to their meat and vegetable products. They added it to make the food taste better to parents, not because it benefited the child. Manufacturers smartly realized that parents commonly taste a baby's food before a feeding.

In 1969, Dr. John Olney at the Washington University School of Medicine in St. Louis found that large amounts of MSG could destroy brain cells in infant mice and monkeys. Though there are differences between newborn mice and 6-month-old babies, the research suggested that as little as four jars of baby food eaten at a time could be dangerous to babies, leaving little margin of safety. In 1969, pressure from Dr. Olney, Ralph Nader, and others persuaded baby-food manufacturers to stop adding MSG to their products.

In the 1970s, pressure from the National Academy of Sciences, American Academy of Pediatrics, and Center for Science in the Public Interest persuaded manufacturers to stop adding salt to baby food. Just as with MSG, salt's primary role was to improve the taste for parents.

Moral of the story? If you're concerned about additives, write to the manufacturers—and ask the FDA to pressure companies to replace questionable additives.

additives that manufacturers had used for decades. The threat keeps growing, too, because Americans' increasing dependence on processed food is causing manufacturers to dump an ever-larger number of chemicals into an ever-larger number of foods.

The children now growing up have been consuming many

questionable additives from birth (and even *in utero*). Their long exposure could make them particularly susceptible to any health problems caused by the additives. Also worrisome is the fact that few additives have been tested for effects on behavior or for interactions with other chemicals with which they might mingle in our children's bodies.

The biggest concern about additives is that some might cause cancer. The National Research Council concluded that additives do "not appear to have contributed to the overall risk of cancer in humans." But it added some important caveats: "This lack of evidence may be due to the relatively recent use of many of these substances," it said, or to the inability of researchers to separate cancers caused by additives from those with other causes. Cancer's long latency period also makes it hard to prove an additive-cancer link, the NRC said.[4]

As the box on page 66 indicates, several commonly used additives have been linked to slightly increased risks of cancer, usually based on animal studies. Those additives include several preservatives—sodium nitrite, BHA, BHT, propyl gallate—and two artificial sweeteners, saccharin and acesulfame-K. While frequent consumption of those additives could be risky, one needn't worry about occasionally eating foods containing them. In fact, because the risks posed to an individual by those additives are quite low, individuals should worry less about being harmed by the additive than about why the FDA permits the continued use of substances that pose even the slightest risk of cancer.

Some dyes and other additives cause allergic reactions. For example, Yellow No. 5—the second most widely used food dye—can cause itching, hives, and headaches. The Food and Drug Administration has estimated that between 47,000 and 94,000 Americans are sensitive to Yellow No. 5.[5]

The medical evidence against Yellow No. 5 is strong enough that Sweden and Norway have banned it. In the United States, the FDA has banned more than 15 dyes after processors used

The Ten Riskiest Food Additives

*O*f the 3,000 chemicals added to food, the following ten additives appear to pose the greatest risk to sensitive individuals and the general population.

Acesulfame-K, a sugar substitute. On the plus side, this and other artificial sweeteners do not promote tooth decay. But acesulfame-K needs lots more tests, because initial trials didn't even meet the FDA's own standards. Those tests, inadequate as they are, indicate that the chemical causes cancer in animals. Acesulfame-K is not yet widely used, but it may be found in some brands of sugar substitutes, chewing gum, dry beverage mixes, instant coffee and tea, gelatin desserts, puddings, and non-dairy creamers. The manufacturer is currently seeking FDA approval for many more uses.

Artificial colorings, used to simulate the presence of fruit or other real ingredients. The government has banned many synthetic dyes over the last few decades, and questions remain about those still used in food. Red No. 3, Yellow No. 5, and other synthetic colors may cause cancer, allergic reactions, or behavioral problems. Manufacturers use dyes in breakfast cereal, candy, ice cream, soft drinks, frostings, and a host of other products.

Aspartame, the most widely used sugar substitute. Several safety questions surround this additive, which is sold commercially as Equal and Nutra-Sweet. Most disturbingly, one test in rats linked aspartame to a slightly higher risk of brain tumors; the test was never repeated. Also, a few consumers have complained of suffering headaches, dizziness, and other problems after consuming foods containing aspartame, though when people who believed they were sensitive to aspartame have been tested in controlled studies, they did not react. Aspartame is widely used in diet soft drinks and other diet foods.

BHA and BHT, two related antioxidants that prevent oils from going rancid. Some tests suggest that both chemicals may be carcinogens. There are lots of safer alternatives. Manufacturers add these preservatives to hundreds of processed foods, including vegetable oil, shortening, potato chips, dry cereals, and bouillon cubes.

Caffeine, a mildly addictive stimulant. Caffeine is the only drug added to the food supply, and children should avoid it as much as possible. Too much caffeine can cause restlessness, nervousness, and insomnia. Caffeine occurs naturally in tea and coffee and is added to Coca-Cola, Pepsi, and many other soft drinks (companies say they add it for its effect on flavor). Letting kids drink a caffeinated beverage at dinner may keep them up into the night, especially if they don't consume caffeine regularly.

Monosodium glutamate (MSG), a flavor enhancer. In some susceptible people MSG causes "Chinese Restaurant Syn-

drome," which is characterized by headaches, tightness in the chest, burning sensations, and other symptoms. Baby-food manufacturers stopped using MSG, but it is still added to a multitude of other processed foods and used by many Chinese restaurants. Hydrolyzed vegetable protein (HVP) is an additive that contains MSG.

Propyl gallate, another antioxidant that is a close cousin of BHA and BHT. One animal study indicated that it caused cancer. As with BHA and BHT, there's no reason propyl gallate should be in our food. It is added to vegetable oil, meat products, potato sticks, chicken soup base, chewing gum, and many other products.

Saccharin, yet another sugar substitute. The FDA tried to ban saccharin in the late 1970s, because the additive caused cancer in laboratory animals. However, because saccharin was then the only artificial sweetener, public and industry outcries

(continued on next page)

(continued from previous page)

persuaded Congress to exempt saccharin from the prohibition against adding cancer-causing chemicals to food. Congress required warning labels instead of the ban. The labels state: "Use of this product may be hazardous to your health. This product contains saccharin, which has been determined to cause cancer in laboratory animals." Saccharin appears most frequently in packets as a substitute for table sugar.

Sodium nitrite, a meat preservative. This chemical can react with other chemicals in food or the body to form tiny amounts of nitrosamines, which are powerful carcinogens. Because nitrosamines form most readily when a food is cooked at high temperature, bacon is the food that is most commonly contaminated. The USDA lowered the permitted levels of nitrite in the 1970s, so this additive is less of a problem than it used to be. Many pro-

cessors are also adding vitamin C or its close (and safe) relative sodium erythorbate to nitrite-containing foods to inhibit the production of nitrosamines. Sodium nitrite is used in most brands of bacon, hot dogs, bologna, ham, and other processed meats, though health-food stores offer nitrite-free alternatives.

Sulfites, a group of preservatives. Sulfites are a danger primarily to the 5 percent to 10 percent of asthmatics who are sulfite-sensitive. Those individuals can have trouble breathing within minutes of eating sulfites, and at least a dozen people are known to have died as a result of consuming the chemical. Congressional pressure has forced the FDA to ban sulfites from most fresh fruits and vegetables, but they still are used in fresh-cut potatoes, dehydrated potatoes, "fresh" shrimp, dried fruits, and wine.

them for years. But Yellow No. 5 remains on the FDA's approved list and is used in candy, soft drinks, ice cream, and many other processed foods.

All dyes would benefit from further testing, but in light of the dyes' miserable safety record, the public would benefit if all of them were banned. Needless to say, manufacturers tremble at such an idea. They contend that color makes food appealing, and they paint a picture of drab inedible-looking food in a world deprived of dyes.

But the truth is natural colorings can often replace synthetic dyes. Those natural colors, derived from beets, peppers, grape skins, saffron, and other sources, are presumably safe (though they haven't been well tested). In fact, processors used natural colorings until chemists developed cheaper, more stable artificial colorings. And many companies who want to call their foods "natural" have been switching back. Most other manufacturers could return to natural colorings, too.

Another fear about additives is that some may cause behavioral problems in children. Dr. Benjamin Feingold grabbed national headlines in the mid-1970s with claims that additives and some natural substances in food were responsible for more than 50 percent of hyperactivity in children. About 2 percent to 4 percent of all children are hyperactive.[6] Many hyperactive children continue to have problems in adulthood. (The term "hyperactivity" has largely been replaced by "attention-deficit hyperactive disorder.")

Numerous studies have tested Dr. Feingold's claims. Many of the tests involved food dyes, because dyes are so widely used, the handful of chemicals was relatively easy to test, and some parents believed dyes were the culprits. About 10 percent of all food eaten in the United States, including many foods targeted at kids, contains artificial colors.[7]

Though much of the medical establishment downplays any link between additives and behavior, several well-designed stud-

Is Your Child Sensitive to Additives?

Every year several children die from allergic reactions to food ingredients. If your child is severely allergic to shellfish, eggs, peanuts, sulfite additives, or other foods or additives, you have to explain very carefully to your child (if he or she can read) how to read labels and avoid the dangerous ingredients. Children with asthma have to be particularly attentive to possible food allergies.

In addition to those severe allergic reactions, certain foods or additives may cause milder allergic or sensitivity (non-immune) reactions. Typical symptoms include nasal congestion, headache, hyperactivity, attention deficits, gas and stomach upset, or other symptoms.

Much of the blame for reactions to foods has focused on additives, but foods themselves are much likelier to cause adverse reactions. The only way to know if your child is sensitive is to eliminate from your child's diet many of the foods and additives that might cause reactions and look for improvements.

According to pediatrician William Crook, author of *Detecting Your Hidden Allergies,* the best approach is to put your child on a one-week special diet. While on this diet, your child *can* eat fresh meat and poultry, any vegetable (except corn, which sometimes causes reactions), fruits and fruit juices (except drinks normally consumed daily), rice, oats, and water. But you must eliminate all of the common allergy-causing foods or chemicals from your child's diet. Those include dairy foods, wheat, eggs, nuts, soybeans, corn products (including corn sugar and syrup), choco-

ies have demonstrated a relationship. For instance, in one Canadian study of 20 hyperactive children, food dyes impaired 17 of 20 hyperactive children in a learning task.[8]

Another carefully controlled study involved 15 boys and 7 girls whose parents felt that food ingredients caused behavioral problems. It was conducted by Bernard Weiss of the University

late, dyes, artificial flavorings, refined sugar, caffeine, BHA, BHT, sodium nitrite, and aspartame.

Dr. Crook recommends feeding your child the limited diet for six or seven days or until you notice two consecutive days of significant improvement. Then add back one of the eliminated foods each day and note in a diary any symptoms that develop. To get a more objective appraisal of your child's behavior, you might ask your child's teacher if he or she notices any change in behavior. But don't tell the teacher that you're changing your child's diet.

Another approach is to feed your child the special diet until you see improvement. Then add back everything over the next couple of days to see if anything in the diet triggers a reaction

If you see a reaction, go back to the special diet and add back foods one by one until you find the foods that cause a problem.

If you have identified foods that cause a problem, have your child avoid them for several weeks and then try them again—cautiously. If the food does not trigger symptoms, consider whether something other than diet may have influenced his or her behavior. It is also possible that your child may be able to eat the food in smaller quantities or infrequently.

In any case, don't expect miraculous changes in symptoms or behavior, because your child might not be sensitive to any ingredient or food at all. And even in kids who react, eliminating the culprits often yields only a partial improvement in symptoms or behavior.

of Rochester School of Medicine and Dentistry and several colleagues in California. One young girl reacted dramatically to dyes and one young boy reacted mildly.[9] Weiss considers that study "a definitive demonstration that, in principle, Feingold was right. That is, some children respond with aberrant behaviors to food dyes delivered at levels encountered in the diet."[10]

Because Weiss's study involved only dyes, additional children might well have reacted to other additives or foods.

A "Consensus Conference" sponsored by the National Institutes of Health in 1982 concluded that while the benefits of an additive-free diet had been exaggerated, it appeared to help some children and might well be given a chance. The panel of experts called for further research.

In 1994, Dr. Bonnie Kaplan and her colleagues at the Alberta (Canada) Children's Hospital reported the effect of diet on 24 hyperactive boys between 3 and 6 years old. This well-designed study involved eliminating from the boys' diets a wide range of ingredients, including artificial colors and flavors, chocolate, monosodium glutamate, preservatives, caffeine, and any substance that families reported might affect their child. According to the researchers, more than half of the children exhibited an improvement in behavior. Some of the children also went to sleep faster and woke up less during the night.[11] The researchers tempered their enthusiasm, though, by noting that none of the children changed overnight into an easy-to-manage person.

Another more recent study (1994) done at the North Shore University Hospital in Manhasset, New York, found similar results in children between the ages of 3 and 11. Dr. Marvin Boris and Dr. Francine S. Mandel found that 19 out of 26 (73 percent) hyperactive children showed improved behavior when artificial colors and preservatives, dairy products, wheat, corn, yeast, soy, citrus, egg, chocolate, and peanuts were eliminated from their diets. When those 19 children were challenged with some of the eliminated foods, all appeared to react to at least three different foods. Sixteen of those children (5 girls, 11 boys) were then secretly fed a suspect food, and all but five had a reaction.

With several studies demonstrating that additives or foods can cause behavioral problems, one might ask why this issue remains mired in controversy. One reason is that manufacturers have deliberately misled the public by pretending that the positive studies don't exist. Also, some of the studies that did not detect any effect did not test large enough amounts of dyes. Sometimes researchers maintained that additives didn't cause problems—even when their own studies indicated otherwise.[13] Finally, the link between additives and behavior is terribly inconvenient to industry. A whole flock of chemical companies would suffer serious financial problems if food manufacturers stopped using additives that affect some children's behavior.

The bottom line is that if your children are displaying behavioral problems, you should test them on an "elimination" diet. The box on pages 70-71 tells you how.

One additive about which there hasn't been *enough* controversy is caffeine, which is present naturally in coffee and tea and added to Coca-Cola, Pepsi, Dr Pepper, Jolt, and other sodas. Caffeine is a stimulant and the only drug added to the food supply.

As many non-coffee drinkers know, an occasional slug of caffeine can keep you up for hours. And as many coffee drinkers know well, going cold turkey on caffeine can cause powerful withdrawal symptoms, which include splitting headaches. Withdrawal symptoms are a clear indication of addictiveness.

Dr. Judith Rapoport, a researcher at the National Institute of Mental Health, and her colleagues have studied the effect of caffeine on grade-school children. Children who consumed large amounts of caffeine—the equivalent of about three cups of coffee or seven cans of Coke a day—were more likely to be nervous, get mad easily, and be more easily frustrated. She also found that among the 30 heaviest consumers of caffeine in a group of 800 children, one out of three "met the criterion for clinical hyperactivity."[14]

In further research, Dr. Rapoport and her colleagues tested the effects of caffeine on boys between about 8 and 12 years old. She gave them amounts of caffeine equivalent to two cups of coffee twice a day. She found that children who normally consumed moderate amounts of caffeine (equivalent to one cup of coffee daily) experienced headache, stomachache, and nausea, and were restless and fidgety and had difficulty going to sleep. Children who normally consumed large amounts of caffeine (equivalent to three cups of coffee daily) apparently had developed a tolerance and experienced fewer side effects.[15]

Parents whose kids never want to go to sleep ought to consider how much caffeine those insomniacs are getting. It's easy to kick soft drinks out of the house (after all, those drinks offer nothing but empty calories); it's even easier to switch to caffeine-free soft drinks.

It simply does not make sense to allow caffeine to be added to beverages consumed in such vast quantities by millions of children. But we suspect that the soft-drink industry, though it denies it, doesn't mind that caffeine is somewhat addictive.

Pesticides

The scary headlines are everywhere: "Watch Those Vegetables, Ma: Pesticide-Laden Produce May Endanger Your Tots," says *Time* magazine. "Are Pesticides Poisoning Our Children?" asks *Woman's Day.* Another *Time* cover asks: "Is Anything Safe?"

If you just skim the headlines, it's easy to believe that poisons lurk in everything you and your children eat. That's not quite the case, but it is a fact that much of the food sold in this country contains pesticide residues. "The average consumer is exposed to pesticide residues, although in minute quantities, in nearly every food, including meat, dairy products, fruits, vegetables, sugar, coffee, oils, dried goods, and most processed foods," said the National Research Council (NRC), an arm of the National Academy of Sciences.[16] Imported produce tends to have higher levels of pesticides than U.S.-grown produce, according to the FDA. Beans, peas, refined sugar, and vegetable oil are among the "cleanest" foods.[17]

American farmers annually apply 700 million pounds[18] of more than 300 different pesticides[19] to crops in order to repel or kill weeds, insects, fungi, bacteria, and rodents. Foreign farmers use another 200 to 300 pesticides on crops,[20] some of which the United States imports.

Fresh fruits and vegetables can get especially large doses of pesticides. "Some are treated a dozen or more times each year with six or more different active ingredients," the NRC said.[21]

The presence of pesticide residues doesn't necessarily make food unsafe. The food industry contends that the tiny amounts of pesticides in food pose no health threat. Unfortunately, in many cases there simply isn't enough hard information to accurately assess whether or not they're right. No one truly knows how much of a health risk pesticides pose to humans. Any risk estimates are, at best, educated guesses.

Nonetheless, some experts have tried to quantify pesticides' risks. For example, the U.S. Environmental Protection Agency rates pesticides as the third greatest cancer risk (after worker exposure to cancer-causing chemicals and radon in homes) among the 29 environmental problems under its jurisdiction. The EPA estimates that pesticides cause cancer in 6,000 Americans annually.[22] In a nation of 250 million people, to a given person that risk is relatively small—but those odds are of no comfort if you or your child happen to be one of those 6,000 people. To put the risk in perspective, the National Research Council says that pesticide residues in food account for only .0025 of a person's risk of developing cancer.[23]

Cancer isn't the only health risk posed by pesticides. "The magnitude of the risk associated with pesticide exposure is just beginning to be understood," Edward Groth, associate technical director at Consumers Union, told a congressional committee in 1991. ". . . [E]vidence is mounting that exposure to pesticide residues in food may have neurotoxic effects and suppress immunity."[24]

Pesticide residues may threaten children far more than they do adults. The reason is twofold. First, relative to their body weight, children eat far more fruits, fruit juices, and possibly other foods than do adults. For example, preschoolers eat six times as much fruit as adults, according to the Natural Resources Defense Council (NRDC), a non-profit environmental group.[25] Eating all this produce exposes children to proportionately higher pesticide levels than adults. The NRDC estimates that as many as 6,200 children may get cancer in their lifetime because of their exposure to eight widely used pesticides.[26] And those eight pesticides are just a fraction of the 66 pesticides that the EPA has identified as potentially carcinogenic.

Apples, apple products, and other foods containing daminozide, or Alar, and its breakdown product, UDMH, posed the greatest cancer risk, said the NRDC. The organization's report *Intolerable Risk: Pesticides in Our Children's Food* triggered a huge controversy over Alar. Ultimately the apple growers stopped using it.

Children also are particularly at risk because their growing bodies may be especially vulnerable to pesticides. "Children are different," said Dr. J. Routt Reigart, a pediatrician who testified before a congressional subcommittee for the American Academy of Pediatrics. "In all sorts of systems as you watch tissues and organs develop and mature, they are much more sensitive than a mature, fully developed organism." Children's metabolism also differs from adults', Dr. Reigart said. That gives children "a tendency to retain chemicals in their system for a longer period of time."[27]

Yet scientists still know little about pesticides' impact on children. ". . . [H]ow children are affected by exposure to chemicals is an evolving science," Linda Fisher, then the U.S.

Pesticide Residues Go Unmeasured

What levels of pesticides lurk in fresh fruits, vegetables, and other foods? Despite reassurances from federal officials, no one really knows.

The Food and Drug Administration is the primary agency charged with testing food for pesticide residues. Unfortunately, its testing program is seriously flawed.

For starters, routine FDA tests can detect only about half the pesticides applied to food. That leaves open the possibility that lots of pesticides slip through undetected. Many of those are cancer-causing fungicides frequently sprayed on fruit, according to the Natural Resources Defense Council's 1989 report, *Intolerable Risk: Pesticides in Our Children's Food.*

Secondly, the FDA tests only a tiny fraction of the nation's food supply. In 1992, for example, the FDA tested only 413 samples of apples across the entire country. It tested just 21 samples of raspberries, 90 samples of watermelon, 78 samples of tomatoes, and 37 samples of eggplant.*

All the problems with the FDA's testing program make its data statistically unreliable, according to the General Accounting Office, the investigative arm of Congress. Without accurate data, it's impossible to determine how safe the nation's food supply really is.†

Since the FDA's pesticide data is so flawed, in 1990 the U.S. Department of Agriculture started its own program to test fruits and vegetables. However, the GAO found that the USDA's program is just as flawed as the FDA's. Just as with the FDA program, the GAO found that the USDA's sampling is statistically unreliable. The net result is that the government still does not accurately know what levels of which pesticides contaminate how much of our food.

---

* "Residue Monitoring 1992," Food and Drug Administration Pesticide Program (1993), 16.

† *Food Safety: USDA Data Program Not Supporting Critical Pesticide Decisions,* U.S. General Accounting Office, GAO/ IMTEC-92-11 (January 1992), 4.

Environmental Protection Agency's top pesticide regulator, told a congressional committee in 1991.[28]

The EPA is responsible for determining what levels of pesticide residues fruits, vegetables, and other foods can legally contain. Based on concerns about how pesticides affect children, you'd think the EPA would consider children's high consumption of fruits and vegetables when setting residue limits. Mostly, though, it does not. "EPA has virtually ignored infant and child food consumption patterns when regulating pesticides," the NRDC concluded in 1989. Instead, the EPA sets residue limits based on adult eating patterns.[29]

Furthermore, the EPA doesn't consider the fact that kids—and adults—frequently ingest several different pesticides at once. "Many foods contain residues of several pesticides," the National Research Council said. "There is no way to know how or whether these interact."[30] The EPA simply ignores those interactions when setting residue limits.

To complicate matters yet further, the EPA set many residue limits decades ago. In the early days of pesticide regulation, the government required few tests. Basically, it rubber-stamped pesticide applications with little proof the pesticide was safe.

Many of these pesticides, especially those registered before 1972, were not tested adequately to see whether they cause either benign or malignant tumors. "Many of these pesticides are widely used today even though some are suspected" of causing tumors, the NRC said.[31] Today the EPA requires manufacturers to conduct fairly rigorous tests of the pesticides' health effects before approving their sale.

Nonetheless, in a 1993 report, *Pesticides in the Diets of Infants and Children,* the National Research Council identified numerous flaws in the way pesticides are regulated and called for sweeping changes. Because of the risks of cancer and other problems, the NRC committee urged the EPA to base pesticide limits "more on health considerations than on agricultural practices."

Moreover, the committee said it is critically important those restrictions be based on children's exposure, not adults'.[32]

The Clinton administration has promised to support legislation that, at long last, would greatly reduce the risks of pesticides in food. As this book went to press, Congress was preparing to grapple with the issue, with industry and environmentalists pressing from opposite directions.

The EPA is also reevaluating the old pesticides to see if they meet current scientific standards. However, it's moving at a snail's pace. The General Accounting Office, the investigative arm of Congress, originally estimated it would take the EPA until 2024 to reregister all the old chemicals. The EPA's slowness angered Congress, so in 1988 it passed a law requiring the agency to finish the job by 1997. EPA isn't going to meet that deadline, though.[33] So, many poorly tested pesticides remain on the market.

How many of them will turn out to be unsafe? There's no way to know for sure. Experience has shown that many pesticides that scientists once considered safe later proved otherwise. In recent years, the EPA has suspended the use of Alar, DDT, dieldrin, heptaclor, kepone, and chlordane because new evidence linked them to health problems.

Defenders of pesticides make light of fears about pesticides' safety. Their standard response to health concerns is simple: Show us someone hurt by pesticides.

Obviously, that's hard to do. Doctors rarely can determine the exact cause of a particular cancer, birth defect, or neurological problem. That's because those health problems may result from a genetic weakness, pollutants, drugs, pesticides, or interactions between any number of substances to which we're exposed. Tumors, after all, aren't labeled with the name of the substance that caused the cancer.

Even when the symptoms of pesticide poisoning are apparent shortly after exposure, it can still be hard to link them to the

Protecting Your Child From Pesticides

While pesticides pose a low health risk compared with high-fat diets, it still makes sense to take precautions that will reduce your child's exposure. When buying and preparing fresh and packaged foods, you can lower your child's pesticide exposure by taking the following steps:

• Thoroughly scrub all produce with a brush. You can add a little dishwashing soap to the water if you like; just be sure to rinse the produce thoroughly after washing. With cauliflower and broccoli, the washing is more effective if you cut up or chop the vegetable first. With leafy vegetables like lettuce and cabbage, throw away the outer leaves and wash the rest.

• Peel apples, peaches, pears, potatoes, and other fruits and vegetables that have skins, since this will remove all surface residues. Peeling lowers the fiber content but the trade-off is worth making as long as your child gets plenty of fiber from other foods.

• Buy as much produce as possible at farmers' markets. Local farmers don't need to douse their fruits and vegetables with post-harvest waxes or pesticides to protect them for a long journey to market.

• Buy certified organic meat, produce, and packaged foods when you can. Those foods are grown and processed without synthetic pesticides. You can buy organic foods at natural-food stores, food cooperatives, farmers' mar-

tainted food. Consider the example of aldicarb. In 1991, aldicarb's manufacturer stopped selling it for use on bananas after bananas were found with ten times the legal residue.[34] Shortly thereafter, EPA officials admitted that even the legal residue was probably unsafe.

Did any child ever get sick from eating a contaminated banana? That's hard to know. The symptoms of aldicarb poisoning are nausea, vomiting, and diarrhea, common to many illnesses. "It would be extremely hard to discern these symptoms from routine childhood illnesses," said Dr. Richard Jack-

kets, by mail, or even at some regular supermarkets. They cost more, but it's worth "voting" for a safer, more environmentally sound approach to agriculture.

• Choose domestically grown produce. Produce from other countries may contain pesticides that the United States has banned. FDA tests find illegal pesticide residues about twice as often in imported produce as in domestic produce. For the same reason, buy produce that is in season. Out-of-season produce is likelier to be grown overseas.

• Don't bypass produce that looks less than perfect. Sometimes, "perfect" produce got that way because it was sprayed with pesticides or waxes. "An awful lot of pesticide use is for cosmetic reasons," said Edward Groth, associate technical director for Consumers Union. Don't buy spoiled or bruised produce, but slightly discolored or misshapen produce is fine.

• If possible, grow your own vegetables. That gives you the ability to choose which, if any, chemicals you use on them. Lettuce, tomatoes, and zucchini are some of the easiest vegetables to grow. Children love to garden and will almost certainly eat the foods they grow.

• Encourage your child to eat a wide variety of produce. This reduces the risk of ingesting a large quantity of a pesticide that may be used on a favorite fruit or vegetable.

son, former chairman of the American Academy of Pediatrics' Committee on Environmental Hazards. "The fact that we haven't had reported much human illness only reflects the fact that we haven't looked for it."[35]

Defenders of pesticides also put the burden of proof on the wrong party. "We are often forced into situations where we are required to prove harm from an agent rather than the producer and user of the agent having to prove safety," Dr. Reigart, the American Academy of Pediatrics spokesman, said in his congressional testimony. "Proving harm is often difficult when the effects, though real, are subtle, occur relatively infrequently, or have a long latency period. We should place the responsibility directly with those responsible for introducing the agents into our environment. We should not force our children to be the guinea pigs that prove after many years that they should not have been exposed."[36]

Perhaps the most frustrating thing about pesticides is that there's no reason for them to contaminate as many foods as they do. David Pimentel, who teaches entomology and agricultural science at Cornell University, estimates that American farmers could reduce their pesticide use by at least 50 percent without any drop in crop yields. "We aren't talking about pie-in-the-sky research to achieve this," Pimentel said. "All the techniques and technologies are already known." Some farmers in both the U.S. and overseas are already using these techniques to farm without any synthetic pesticides at all.

Other countries have begun reducing their reliance on pesticides. Both Sweden and Denmark have developed programs to reduce pesticide use 50 percent by the mid- to late 1990s. The Netherlands is working on a similar plan.[37]

Why are American farmers lagging behind? There are many reasons, Pimentel said, including the fact that both federal price-support programs and advertising by pesticide manufacturers encourage heavy use of chemicals. "We don't have sufficient incentives in place to encourage farmers to substitute non-chemical controls for chemical controls," Pimentel said.

Replacing half of all pesticides with safer means of pest control would cost about $1 billion annually, Pimentel and his colleagues estimate, which could push up food prices by 0.6 percent. That's a tiny price to pay for safer food and a cleaner environment.[38]

Whether they like it or not, American farmers may be quickly approaching the day when they have to embrace alternative methods for controlling pests. That's because while pesticide use keeps climbing, pesticide effectiveness keeps falling. Pimentel and his colleagues found that pesticide use has risen 33-fold in the United States since 1945. Yet over the same period, the dollar value of crops lost to pests rose from 31 percent to 37 percent.[39]

Why did crop losses rise during the same period that pesticide use skyrocketed? Largely because many farmers stopped rotating crops and instead continuously planted the same crop in the same field, Pimentel said. Heavy pesticide use also destroyed many natural enemies of pests, he said, and lots of pests grew resistant to pesticides.

Pimentel predicts that within the next five to ten years, public pressure will force American farmers to reduce their use of pesticides. During that same period, the EPA may finally make progress in reevaluating old pesticides and banning those that threaten health. Also, in 1995 a law is expected to go into effect that will provide the first national definition of "organic" food, giving organic farming the credibility that it deserves.

Those developments will reduce the threat posed by pesticides, but they're years away. In the meantime, all the bad publicity about pesticides on produce might tempt you to eliminate fruits and vegetables from your children's diets. But doing so would be a serious mistake. According to Dr. Jackson, "A diet rich in fruits and vegetables accounts for profound human health benefits both in terms of heart disease and cancer prevention. The benefits of a diet rich in fruits and vegetables greatly outweigh the risks."[40]

Clearly, feeding your kids natural foods carries some risk. Based on current knowledge, though, that risk is relatively small. By contrast, the risk associated with *not* feeding your kids produce and other natural foods is high. By taking the few precautions outlined in the box, "Protecting Your Child from Pesticides," on pages 80–81, you can protect your kids while also letting them revel in the tastes—and the benefits—of fresh fruits, vegetables, low-fat milk, and other natural foods.

CHAPTER 5

Eat Your Veggies… and Other Good Foods

D espite the gloomy picture presented in the preceding chapters—the bad news about the quantities of fat, sugar, and salt in kids' food; the rising incidence of childhood obesity; and the risks bacteria, pesticides, and additives present—there is a brighter side to the story. Eating enough vegetables, fruits, and other nutrient-packed foods can enhance your health, and may actually help prevent certain diseases, including cancer.

In fact, people who eat diets rich in fruit and vegetables (including beans) appear to have lower risks of cancers of the lung, colon, stomach, mouth, throat, rectum, and bladder. The National Cancer Institute (NCI) urges all Americans to eat at least five servings of fruit and vegetables each day. Younger children should eat smaller servings, but they should still try for "five a day." Unfortunately, this doesn't seem to be happening. The U.S. Department of Agriculture did a survey and found that on that day 30 percent of elementary school children and about 60 percent of teenagers had eaten no fruit at all.[1] An NCI study found that at least one in four children in elementary and high school does not even eat one serving of vegetables (not counting French fries) per day.[2]

What constituent[s] in fruit and vegetables act to prevent disease? Researchers aren't sure. It could be:

• **Carotenes and/or vitamin C.** Carotenes give cantaloupe, carrots, sweet potatoes, and other foods their orange color. The body turns one form, called beta-carotene, into vitamin A. People who eat foods rich in beta-carotene, as opposed to liver and other foods rich in vitamin A itself, have a lower risk of several cancers.

Some researchers believe beta-carotene may protect against cancer because it's an antioxidant. Chemicals with antioxidant properties may prevent oxygen and other chemicals from damaging cells. Other studies suggest that foods rich in vitamin C— another antioxidant—also reduce the risk of cancer.

Scientists are doing many more studies on beta-carotene and vitamin C. But you needn't wait for the results to encourage your children to eat foods that contain them. Among the best: sweet potatoes, carrots, cantaloupe, mangos, oranges, spinach and other greens, broccoli, apricots, and red peppers.

• **Fiber.** Fruits, vegetables, beans, and whole grains are rich in dietary fiber. Fiber helps move food through the large intestine, reducing the risk of constipation. Fiber-rich foods may also reduce the risk of colon and rectum cancers.

A major study on diet and cancer in men provided strong evidence that high-fiber diets protect against cancers of the colon and rectum. Men who consumed more than 28 grams of dietary fiber daily had one-third the risk for colorectal cancer than

Virtuous Vegetables

*A*ll vegetables are fine to eat, but some have more nutri-ents than others. This chart rates the most common vegetables according to their nutritional content. The scores add up the Daily Value of six nutrients commonly found in vegetables (beta-carotene, vitamin C, folate, iron, copper, calcium) plus dietary fiber. Thus, a serving of vegetable containing 50 percent of the Daily Value for vitamin C and 10 percent of the Daily Value for calcium would have a score of 60.

VEGETABLE (½ cup cooked, unless noted)	SCORE
Sweet potato, no skin *(1)*	582
Carrot, raw *(1)*	434
Carrots	408
Spinach	241
Collard greens	181
Red pepper	166
Kale	161
Dandelion greens	156
Spinach, raw *(1 cup)*	152
Broccoli	145
Brussels sprouts	128
Potato, baked, w/skin *(1)*	114
Mixed vegetables, frozen	111
Winter squash	110
Swiss chard	105
Snow peas	90
Mustard greens	85
Kohlrabi	82

men who consumed under 17 grams.[3]

Although scientists aren't sure how dietary fiber might pro-tect against cancer, some think that by adding bulk to stools fiber lowers the concentration of cancer-causing substances that come in contact with the walls of the intestine.

American children ages 4 to 19 eat an average of only 12 grams of fiber daily.[4] The NCI reports that in countries where people eat twice that amount, the rates of colon and rectal can-cers are lower than in the United States.[5] Those two cancers kill a total of almost 60,000 Americans each year. The NCI recom-

Romaine lettuce *(1 cup)*	78		Boston lettuce *(1 cup)*	38
Cauliflower	77		Green beans	37
Cauliflower, raw	77		Tomato *(½)*	37
Asparagus	75		Beets	32
Green peppers *(½)*	67		Summer squash	31
Potato, baked, no skin *(1)*	67		Onions	27
Parsley *(¼ cup)*	66		Green beans, canned	26
Green peas, frozen	64		Turnips	26
Avocado, California *(½)*	63		Lettuce, leaf *(1 cup)*	25
Okra	61		Lettuce, iceberg *(1 cup)*	22
Collard greens	57		Radishes *(¼ cup)*	17
Endive, raw *(1 cup)*	56		Celery (1 stalk)	14
Parsnips	53		Onions *(¼ cup)*	14
Rutabaga	48		Eggplant	12
Cabbage	47		Alfalfa sprouts *(½ cup)*	11
Artichoke *(½)*	46		Cucumber	11
Mushrooms	43		Mushrooms	10
Cabbage, raw	39		Garlic *(1 clove)*	3
Corn	39			

Source: *Nutrition Action Healthletter,* December, 1991, p. 11.

mends that everyone over age 2 eat 20 to 30 grams of fiber daily.[6] Thus, most children—and adults—need to double their fiber consumption.

To increase your children's fiber intake, serve more fruits, vegetables, whole-grain breads, cereals, grains, pasta, and cooked dry peas and beans. Some especially good sources of fiber include bran cereal, whole-wheat spaghetti, beans (for example, pinto, garbanzo, black), lentils, green peas, corn, potatoes (with skin), sweet potatoes, carrots, apples, pears, strawberries, oranges, and bananas.

• **Other plant constituents.** It's possible that something other than (or in addition to) the vitamins or dietary fiber in fruits and vegetables reduces the risk of cancer. More and more research suggests that phytochemicals, or plant chemicals, are highly beneficial. Phytochemicals have exotic-sounding names, like flavonoids, polyacetylenes, lignans, and isoflavones. Varying amounts of different phytochemicals are present in every fruit, grain, and vegetable. In animal studies, some of them seem to protect against tumors, but it's too early to say for sure that they have the same effect in people.[7]

• **Low fat intake.** Throughout the world, the populations that eat more fruit, vegetables, beans, and whole grains also eat less fat. Many scientists think that both the smaller amount of fat and the larger amount of plant foods account for the lower cancer risk.

If you're cutting your child's fat intake only by replacing red meat with fish, whole milk with skim milk, and fatty sweets (cakes, cookies, ice cream, etc.) with fat-free versions, you've made important changes, but need to take additional steps. Most experts agree that the typical American diet is too rich in animal foods—even low-fat foods like skinless chicken and skim milk—and too low in plant foods. Both adults and children need to shift that balance in favor of plants.

That scares many parents who fear that without a lot of animal foods their children will develop protein deficiencies. Not true. The incidence of protein deficiency among American children is nil.

If anything, the nutrients in animal foods that kids may run short on are zinc and iron (found in meat, fish, and poultry) and calcium (found in many dairy products). But you can also find these nutrients in plant foods. Good sources include:

• Zinc: beans, wheat germ, tofu, chicken breast.
• Iron: green leafy vegetables, legume beans, bulgur.

Fabulous Fruits

*F*ruits are among most kids' favorite foods. In addition to sweetness, fruits provide a variety of vitamins, minerals, and other goodies. To rate fruits, we added up the Daily Values of nine valuable nutrients—beta-carotene, vitamin C, folate, thiamin, riboflavin, niacin, potassium, iron, calcium—plus fiber.

FRUIT (serving size)	SCORE
Papaya (½)	252
Cantaloupe (¼)	213
Strawberries (1 cup)	186
Orange (1)	169
Tangerines (2)	168
Kiwi (1)	154
Mango (½)	153
Apricots (4)	143
Persimmon (1)	134
Watermelon (2 cups)	122
Raspberries (1 cup)	117
Grapefruit (red or pink) (½)	103
Blackberries (1 cup)	101
Apricots, dried (10)	97
Grapefruit, white (½)	84
Honeydew melon (⅒)	81
Peaches (2)	77
Pineapple (1 cup)	77
Star fruit (1)	73
Blueberries (1 cup)	68
Cherries, sweet (1 cup)	64
Nectarine (1)	64
Pomegranate (1)	61
Banana (1)	60
Plums (2)	60
Prunes, dried (5)	59
Apple, with skin (1)	58
Boysenberries (1 cup)	57
Pear (1)	48
Grapes, green (60)	46
Peaches, canned in juice (2 slices)	43
Apple, no skin (1)	42
Pineapple, canned in juice (2 slices)	40
Figs, dried (2)	39
Currants, dried (¼ cup)	36
Rhubarb, cooked (½ cup)	36
Raisins (¼ cup, packed)	35
Dates (5)	30
Pears, canned in juice (2 halves)	16

Source: *Nutrition Action Healthletter,* May, 1992, p. 11.

Best Beans

*B*eans *are generally low-fat sources of protein, dietary fiber, and various vitamins and minerals. This chart rates the nutritional values of the most common beans according to their content of folate, magnesium, potassium, iron, copper, zinc, and protein, plus dietary fiber. The scores are obtained by adding up the Daily Values for those nutrients. (The scoring system is not complete: Beans contain many more than seven nutrients.) If a one-cup serving of beans provides at least 50 percent of the Daily Value of any nutrients, those are listed.*

BEAN (1 cup, cooked)	SCORE	ABUNDANT NUTRIENTS
Soybeans	300	iron
Pinto beans	287	fiber, folate
Chickpeas (garbanzos)	286	fiber, folate
Lentils	285	fiber, folate
Cranberry beans	278	fiber, folate
Black-eyed peas (cowpeas)	273	folate
Pink beans	269	folate
Navy beans	266	fiber, folate
Black beans (turtle beans)	265	fiber, folate
Small white beans	263	fiber, folate
White beans	253	
Lima beans, baby	252	fiber, folate
Kidney beans, all types	243	folate
Adzuki beans	238	folate
Great Northern beans	228	fiber
Broadbeans (fava beans)	197	
Peas, split (green)	192	fiber
Tofu, raw, firm (4 oz.)	178	iron
Tofu, raw, regular (4 oz.)	109	

Source: *Nutrition Action Healthletter,* May, 1993, p. 13.

Great Grains

*B*read, rice, pasta, and other foods made from grains should provide a large percentage of children's calories. Grains are naturally low in fat and high in fiber. The scores shown here add up the Daily Values for five nutrients (magnesium, zinc, copper, iron, vitamin B_6) plus dietary fiber. For instance, a grain with 15 percent of the Daily Value for zinc and 10 percent for iron would have a score of 25.

GRAIN (5 ounces, cooked)	SCORE
Quinoa	73
Macaroni or spaghetti (whole wheat)	69
Amaranth	66
Buckwheat groats (kasha)	64
Spaghetti (spinach-flavored)	61
Bulgur	60
Barley, pearled	59
Wild rice	58
Millet	53
Brown rice	51
Triticale	47
Spaghetti	42
Wheat berries	41
Kamut	37
Oats, rolled	33
Spelt	33
White rice, converted	26
Couscous	23
White rice, instant	18
Soba noodles	12
Corn grits	10

Source: *Nutrition Action Healthletter*, April, 1993, p. 11.

- Calcium: tofu made with calcium sulfate, collard and turnip greens, kale, broccoli.

And no one's saying you have to eliminate *all* animal foods from your child's diet. According to the U.S. Department of Agriculture, reasonable daily targets are:

- 6 to 11 servings of bread (2 slices), cereal (1 cup; ½ cup of granola), rice (¾ cup), and pasta (1 cup).

- 4 to 6 servings of vegetables (1 cup leafy greens; ½ cup cooked or raw) and beans (½ cup cooked).
- 2 to 4 servings of fruits or fruit juice (1 cup).
- 2 to 3 servings of milk or yogurt (1 cup), cheese (1 ounce), and cottage cheese (½ cup).
- 1 to 2 servings of fish, poultry, meat (4 ounces, cooked), nuts (¼ cup), peanut butter (2 tablespoons), and eggs (1).

The smaller number of servings—and smaller serving sizes—are more appropriate for young children. The larger numbers of servings are appropriate for older kids, especially teenage boys. Kids ages 11 and older need three servings of dairy products or other calcium-rich foods to get their Recommended Dietary Allowance for calcium (1,200 milligrams).

Of course, cancer is not the only thing that vegetables, fruits, grains, and beans are good at fighting, especially as your children grow older. For instance, the dietary fiber prevents constipation, the folic acid reduces the risk of certain birth defects, and the calcium helps prevent osteoporosis (brittle bones). Our bottom line is to fill up your kids on a variety of vegetable-based products; they offer a wealth of health benefits and an incredible variety of tastes. (If you are concerned about avoiding pesticide contamination, please see "Protecting Your Child From Pesticides," pages 80–81.)

PART 2

Why Kids Eat the Way They Do

CHAPTER 6

How Food Companies Seduce Kids

A s a quick introduction to the world of marketing to kids, let's take a look at a day in the life of a hypothetical 8-year-old girl—we'll call her Amy.

While Amy gobbles down her Teenage Mutant Ninja Turtles cereal at breakfast, she plays with the plastic McDonald's restaurant that Mattel created for Barbie. Barbie's sister, Skipper, visits the restaurant wearing an outfit plastered with Pepsi logos.

Then it's off to school. Amy's teacher uses the Environmental Action Pack, created by McDonald's, to teach a lesson about ecology. Amy and her classmates make food-chain wheels, learn about problems with trash, and start their own recycling projects. All the activity sheets Amy's teacher copied for the students carry the McDonald's logo. The Environmental Action Pack is one of more than two dozen educational items McDonald's sells to teachers.

Seeing that McDonald's logo everywhere can make a little girl hungry, but Amy's in luck: It's time for lunch. In the school cafeteria, Amy gets to choose among hamburgers, pizza, deep-fried chicken nuggets, french fries, and other favorite foods. In lots of school cafeterias, it's hard to tell you're not in a fast-food restaurant. That's because officials at some schools think that cafeterias can only succeed financially if they serve kids the same kind of food as McDonald's, Taco Bell, and Pizza Hut.

After lunch, it's back to class to listen to a guest speaker. She's a volunteer from the local Burger King who's speaking as part of BK's "Adopt A School" program. While she's there, she presents awards to Amy and other outstanding students.

The big event, though, comes during the last hour of school. That's when Pizza Hut delivers enough pizzas for the whole class. The party, part of Pizza Hut's "Book It!" program, rewards the students for reading a certain number of books. Amy and her classmates also get certificates good for free pizzas.

Back at home again, Amy flips on the TV and watches cartoons: Disney's *Gummi Bears, Teenage Mutant Ninja Turtles,* and *Tiny Toons Adventures.* It's hard for her to separate the shows from commercials. That's because *Gummi Bears* was spun off from a candy; *Teenage Mutant Ninja Turtles* has scores of licensed products, including Turtles Cereal, Turtles Fruit Snacks, Chef Boyardee Turtles pasta, and many other foods; and *Tiny Toons Adventures* also shows up as a cereal. While she watches, she munches on Garfield and Friends Chewy Fruit Snacks. Never mind that they contain virtually no fruit.

Amy sees dozens of commercials. Most push fast food, sugared cereals, and candy. Amy particularly enjoys the McDonald's ads, since she's playing with her McDonald's Cooking Center as she watches TV. The Cooking Center, produced by Fisher-Price, has a pretend fry warmer, a deep fryer, and a grill. For her birthday, maybe Amy will get the McDonald's Soda Fountain to make her restaurant complete. For added realism, Amy dresses in her McDonald's Crew Uniform by Fisher-Price.

Amy tires of playing, so she lies down to read her newsletter from the Burger King Kids Club. The newsletter conveniently lists upcoming premiums at Burger King and contains lots of ads for Pepsi, Sega, and other products. Amy plots out future visits to the restaurant.

Amy's mother invites several of Amy's friends over for dinner. They crowd around the table to choose between Franco-American's Garfield PizzOs and 'Where's Waldo SpaghettiOs. The girls zap their dinners, and top them off with Teenage Mutant Ninja Turtles sandwich cookies for dessert.

After dinner, they turn on the Nintendo game and slap in the cartridge for Spot: The Video Game. The game features the character from 7Up ads breakdancing, diving, and moonwalking.

The girls start dancing around, imitating Spot and recreating 7Up ads. That leads them to start playing Adverteasing Junior. It's a board game where players advance by recalling slogans and jingles from ads for fast foods, cereals, toys, and cartoons.

Tired by the game, the girls plop in front of the TV to watch a movie. What will it be? Try their thirty-third viewing of *Teenage Mutant Ninja Turtles*. The movie features Domino's Pizza, Pepsi, and Burger King, all included as a result of marketing deals. The food references make the girls hungry again. They get out Amy's Domino's Pizza oven—a toy version that really bakes—and cook mini pizzas from mixes. To wash down the pizza, they grab bottles of 7Up and Pepsi from the fridge.

After Amy's friends leave, she crawls into bed between her Ninja Turtles sheets. As she drifts off to sleep, Amy starts dreaming of the day when she'll grow up and go off to college. Maybe, if she's really lucky, she'll get to study fast-food marketing at Washington State University with the Taco Bell distinguished professor. Taco Bell got the professorship named after it by giving WSU a $250,000 endowment.[1]

Forget whatever you learned about childhood being a carefree time of innocent pleasures. Today, marketers grab children when they're barely able to walk and talk in order to indoctrinate them with messages to buy, buy, buy. It's little wonder that in some families, a child's first sentence is "Go McDonald's."

Selling to kids is big business, and few are better at it than the food companies. Their tools range from "educational" materials prepared for schools to kids clubs to massive television advertising campaigns.

Why all the focus on kids? Because they represent big bucks. Long gone are the days when kids considered themselves lucky if they got a quarter a week in allowance. Today, the 72 million Americans age 19 and below spend billions of dollars each year.

James McNeal, a marketing professor at Texas A&M University, estimates that kids ages 4 to 12 had a total income of $14.3 billion in 1991 and an average weekly income per child of $8.13. They spent $8.5 billion of that money, with more than one-third going for food and beverages.[2] The estimates of how much 13-to-19-year-olds spend vary widely, but $60 billion to $70 billion is plausible. Some analysts claim the average adolescent now spends well over $2,000 annually, more than twice as much as a decade ago.[3]

With millions of kids having billions of dollars in their pockets, is it any wonder that food marketers target children virtually from birth? Michael Evans, a Burger King spokesman, happily tells of a brand-new father who stopped at Burger King right after leaving the hospital to sign up his baby for the Kids Club. The baby's name and address went in the company's database, and he'll get targeted mailings for years. It's a marketer's dream come true.

Besides spending billions themselves, kids also influence many more billions in family purchases of everything from breakfast cereals to personal computers. McNeal estimates that kids ages 4 to 12 influence slightly more than $128 billion in household purchases annually. Others estimate that kids ages 12 to 17 guide more than $150 billion in family spending.[4] If you stir around the two numbers and throw in a few billion extra for purchases swayed by kids below age 4, you have $300 billion or so in annual household spending influenced by children.

In the old days, marketers just targeted children with ads for traditional kids' products like toys and candy. Today, marketers are increasingly promoting to children products that aren't child-oriented, said Dale Kunkel, assistant professor of communications at the University of California–Santa Barbara. "Advertisers are beginning to appreciate the potential for influencing children to influence their parents on a lot of general family purchases," Kunkel said.

Kids' influence is particularly strong on food purchases. That's at least partly because it usually costs a parent little to comply with a child's request. Parents may not let their children choose the family's new car, but they may let them pick a frozen pizza or the restaurant where the family eats. McNeal says that food accounts for nearly $80 billion of the $128 billion in family purchases that 4-to-12-year-olds influence.

Somewhere between 60 percent and 90 percent of teens buy groceries for their families (depending on whose survey you believe[5]) giving them a direct impact on food purchases. Teen food shoppers are particularly common in families with only one parent or where both parents work. No one knows how much teens spend at grocery stores, but it's surely in the tens of billions of dollars.

Marketers virtually drool over the billions that kids spend directly or indirectly. "Throughout the world, children are changing fast from kids to consumers," states *Fortune.* "Savvy marketers are both capitalizing on the trend and speeding it along."[6] No point letting kids be kids, now is there? Not according to Ann Clurman, senior vice president at the market research firm Yankelovich Clancy Shulman. "Children are consumers-in-training," she told *Marketing & Media Decisions.*[7]

An article headlined "Picking Junior's Pocket" in *The Marketer* describes how direct-mail marketers can hook kids. "Today's kids have cash in their pockets, Nintendo on the brain, and guilt-tripped parents buying them almost anything," it proclaims. "To direct marketers, this is nirvana."[8] Indeed.

Marketers Invade Little Leagues

Kids can't even play baseball in the summer without food marketers butting in. In 1991, Leaf Inc., maker of PayDay and Heath bars, Milk Duds, Good & Plenty, Jolly Rancher, and other candies, sent a letter to 60,000 youth baseball coaches and league presidents nationwide. The pitch: If your kids collect wrappers from our candy, we'll send you free equipment. Leaf offered jerseys, baseballs, bats, pitching machines, and other equipment—20 cents' worth for each wrapper collected.

The targeted coaches worked with 1.5 million kids. Numbers like that could translate into sales of lots of candy bars. Some youth-league concession stands started carrying Leaf products because of the wrapper promotion, according to *Adweek's Marketing Week.**

"If it encourages kids to eat our candy versus another candy bar, you can say this is marketing in a cynical fashion," says Michael McIntyre, Leaf's sports marketing manager. "But I tend to look at it in more of a positive vein, that we are doing a service to the local community and to the kids."

The Leaf program has some good points, the most important being that kids get something worthwhile from it. But it has lots of nutritional negatives. It pushes kids to eat candy not because they want it but for its wrapper. The qualities of the food itself become irrelevant.

It also enlists coaches—who ought to be promoting healthful lifestyles—to spur them on. If, for instance, Coach says the team needs 200 wrappers for a case of baseballs, what child can resist feeling compelled to bring in his or her share?

---

*Fara Warner, "Leaf Joins Little League," *Adweek's Marketing Week,* April 22, 1991, 8.

The article provides helpful tips on preparing a direct-mail package that kids will find irresistible. It states: "The winners usually have three elements: some sort of social redemption, meaning the marketer has to disguise its intentions of merely peddling goods to children; kind-and-quick service; and an inviting, easily readable package."

Marketers are targeting kids at ever-younger ages. Some researchers believe that kids can develop brand loyalties as early as age 9 and often probably much earlier.[9] Brand loyalty is a holy concept to marketers. They know that if they can get a child to eat Toasty Woasties, the child might buy the cereal for the rest of his or her life. That makes it imperative to snare their devotion early. Never mind that children don't understand the persuasive intent of advertising until at least age 7 or 8.[10]

To hook kids on their brands, food and beverage marketers are using an increasingly broad array of devices. As Amy's day began to illustrate, some of the most popular tools include kids clubs, tie-ins with popular movies or TV shows, product placements in movies, premiums, toys and clothes tied into a brand-name food, and razzle-dazzle TV commercials. In the rest of this chapter, we'll examine all of these devices except TV commercials. The commercials deserve a whole chapter of their own, so we'll look at them in Chapter 7.

Kids Clubs

Burger King has virtually written the book on how to run a successful kids club. During the 1980s, the company pretty much conceded the children's market to McDonald's, the industry leader in fast food. Burger King didn't even advertise on Saturday-morning TV.

That all changed January 1, 1990, when Burger King

launched its Kids Club. The company set a goal of attracting one million members by the end of the year. To Burger King's surprise and joy, by August 1990 the club had two million. By December 1993, it had four million. "This has been a great vehicle for us," said Michael Evans, manager of media relations for Burger King.[11]

Why the sudden focus on kids? "Because studies have shown that children in the 4-to-9 age group have a tremendous impact on the purchasing decisions when it comes to fast food," said Evans. Indeed they do. In a Roper Poll done for *USA Weekend*, 78 percent of parents said their kids influence where they go for fast food.[12] Some 1.7 million kids under age 6 eat at fast-food restaurants each day, according to *The Wall Street Journal*.[13]

"What we're trying to do is add value and extend the experience," Evans said. "Traditionally, you go into a fast-food restaurant, you buy your meal, you get your toy, you eat, you go home, and that's it. What we're trying to do is to build a little bit more of a relationship with these young people."

The "leaders" of the Kids Club are cartoon characters with names like Kid Vid, I.Q., Wheels, Jaws, Snaps, and Boomer. "It's sort of like a nineties Spanky and Our Gang kind of thing," explained Evans.

The Kids Club targets 4-to-12-year-olds. They can sign up for free at any Burger King by filling out a form that asks for their name, address, birth date, and sex. A massive computer database gobbles up all the information. A few weeks after signing up, kids get their Super Official Totally Secret Membership Kit in the mail. It includes a membership card, a page of Kids Club stickers, a small poster featuring the Kids Club characters, and offers from TWA and *World Book Encyclopedia.*

Evans denied that the Kids Club is simply a cynical marketing ploy that gives kids little of value. "I think we've taken a very responsible approach," he said. "We do not sell [the kids' names] to other companies. If we would, that database would be worth—you couldn't imagine. Although we do direct-mail efforts, we don't inundate them," Evans said, adding that the newsletters and a booklet that Burger King provides have "legitimate educational and fun activities to stimulate the children."

Anyone who reads the newsletter, called *Adventure,* might contest Evans' claims about its alleged virtues. Kids pick up the newsletter when they visit Burger King. Highlights from a typical issue include the following:

- A front-page drawing of *The Simpsons,* one of Burger King's key licensing tie-ins, along with a note urging kids to watch the show.
- A song set to the tune of "Three Blind Mice" that tells kids not to litter.
- A "sneak peak" at *The Simpsons* collectible toys soon to be available at Burger King. The copy encourages kids to collect all five—at $3.49 each.
- A letter from a 5-year-old Kids Club member describing the "blast" she had during her birthday party at Burger King. Kid Vid responds by explaining how other kids can have their birthday parties at Burger King, too.

In the four-page newsletter, "Burger King" appears 20 times. In another issue, the name appears 19 times.

In fairness, the newsletter does possess a few socially redeeming qualities. For example, it portrays handicapped children in a positive light. The character Wheels is a handicapped boy who uses a wheelchair.

Mostly, though, the booklet pushes kids to keep going back to Burger King. One method is a contest that requires kids to check for their name and membership number on a chart at Burger King. If they match, they win a cardboard Kids Club Clubhouse. The booklet urges kids to keep checking for their names because "there'll be up to 100 new winners and awesome new prizes almost every month." In any given month, the odds of winning are less than one in 27,000.

Why is the Kids Club so successful? Evans thinks it's partly because kids like to get mail. "The ongoing program allows them to look for the newest edition of the newsletter, to write letters in, to submit photographs of their families, and to take an active role in this organization," Evans said.

It's certainly debatable whether letting kids send in letters and pictures, only a few of which Burger King publishes in the newsletter or booklet, truly gives them an "active role." In truth, their only "active role" is to keep running to Burger King.

Peggy Charren, founder of Action for Children's Television (which closed in 1992), said this lack of a "meaningful relationship" between kids and a club is common. She also finds little value in the mailings that clubs send to members. "Most of the stuff they send them in the mail is connections to other products or to the product they're pushing in the first place," Charren said.

While joining Burger King's club is free, membership in Kraft's now-defunct Cheese & Macaroni Club cost $2.95 and three proofs of purchase from Kraft General Foods products. For their money, kids got a wrist pouch, a bike license plate, plastic sunglasses, a membership card, a certificate, and a "Fun Book with great Club stuff to order later." To push the club, in 1991 Kraft automatically entered new members into a sweepstakes for a Sega Genesis video-game system.

The club was "a fun activity for kids whose parents are our most loyal consumers," said Nancy Nevin, communications manager for Kraft General Foods. The club, which started in 1990, had 32,000 members by June 1991.

The entire "activity" of the club consisted of Kraft sending kids mailings a couple of times a year. Nevin said the mailings typically consisted of a Fun Book and a premium, such as sunglasses or a bracelet. "It's not designed to be an interactive type of thing," she said of the club. "Kids like to get mail. It's just one way to reach out to them and make them feel like they're kind of a special part of the family because they get mail, too."

The Fun Book sent to new members opens with three letters from kids extolling the club and Kraft Macaroni & Cheese. "I eat Kraft Macaroni and Cheese almost every day of the week," wrote one child. "It's good. By the way, thank you for everything you gave me since I've joined. There's only one food that I really like, that's Kraft Macaroni and Cheese."

Two of the Fun Book's eight pages push merchandise emblazoned with "Kraft Cheese & Macaroni Club." The rest of the book consists primarily of puzzles and pictures that include Kraft characters or products. The Cheese & Macaroni Club was replaced in 1992 by other child-oriented promotions.

Was the club simply a marketing gimmick? "I don't consider this to be a gimmick at all," Nevin said. She added that Kraft won't sell its membership list to other marketers.

Kraft General Foods also dominates the Fox Kids Club, run by the Fox Television Network. The club's magazine, *Totally Kids,* is basically a 12-page, full-color ad for Kraft General Foods products.

For example, there's a full-page ad for Cool Whip. The ad includes three "recipes" for snacks kids can make. One, for "Cookie Pizza Pie," instructs kids to spread Cool Whip on a cookie, sprinkle on shredded coconut, and then top the whole mess with red and green candies.

Many other companies also sponsor kids clubs. There's the Nickelodeon Club, the Mickey Mouse Club, and the MTV Record Club, to name a few. Although food companies don't run these clubs, there is often a food tie-in. For example, Nickelodeon launched its club through Pizza Hut, and the Fox Kids Club magazine runs ads for the Burger King Kids Club (as well as for Kraft products). The Mickey Mouse Club takes food marketing full circle. Boxes of Mickey's Parade Ice Cream Treats have order forms so kids can join, and the club sends them coupons for M&M's, Denny's restaurants, and Hi-C drinks.

Consumers Union, publisher of *Consumer Reports* magazine, charged that kids clubs are a "cause for concern" because of their power over kids. "Clubs disguise commercial messages," a CU report concluded. "Kids are invited to join something that promises to be 'theirs,' but turns out to be a way of manipulating them to buy things. The ad messages come disguised as 'advice from your club,' making them more difficult to resist. The more a child's guard is down, the more effective an ad can be."

Nonetheless, James McNeal—the Texas A&M marketing professor—predicts that clubs are the wave of the future. "With the rapid appearance of database marketing, the two just fit together very well," he said. Peggy Charren agrees. "Anything that makes money for manufacturers and advertisers will continue until we have a federal government that stops them from using manipulative, deceptive, and illegal practices," she said. "The profit system is an incredible incentive to manipulate children unless we move in and moderate it."

Tie-ins

How did Burger King attract millions of kids to its restaurants to sign up for the Kids Club? The company didn't tout its burgers. Burger King had something a lot better than fast food: It had the Teenage Mutant Ninja Turtles.

Just as the Kids Club started, Burger King offered Turtles badges in its Kids Meals. Turtles mania was growing at a frantic pace, and Burger King handed out nearly 15 million Turtles badges in just six weeks.[14]

Only a few weeks later, Burger King started offering Turtles videos for $3.49 with any meal purchase. Within weeks, the

Is the Gum French-Fry Flavored?

In 1990, Canada Post Corporation printed McDonald's arches in the margins around sheets of stamps aimed at children. The stamps pictured mythological creatures, including bigfoot, a werewolf, and two sea monsters. Canada Post designed the stamps to attract kids to stamp collecting.

That they probably did. But they also served as an unusual advertising message for McDonald's—one that carried the implied seal of approval of the Canadian government.

In 1992, another food company, Kraft General Foods, was the "official sponsor" of Canada's Olympic stamp booklet. As with the McDonald's issue, the Kraft logo appeared in the sheet margins.

Both McDonald's and Kraft paid sponsorship fees.

Brenda Adams, media relations manager for Canada Post, declined to say how much the companies paid.

Adams sees nothing wrong with printing corporate logos on sheet margins. "The sponsorship itself is not an endorsement of a company's products," she said. Doesn't it at least imply an endorsement? "I don't know," she said. "I think what it does is it simply shows a relationship or partnership between the two organizations." That may be a bit too subtle for most kids to comprehend.

Ultimately, what the stamps teach kids about Canada is that if you have enough money, you can even buy advertising space on stamps issued by the government. That's hardly a positive lesson.

restaurant chain was reportedly selling about 200,000 videos every day.[15] With Burger King offering a different Turtles video each week for four weeks, kids had a powerful incentive to keep going back.

The crime-fighting, pizza-loving Turtles are a marketing phenomenon unparalleled in recent history. Marketers of every size, shape, and description have plastered them on everything from kids' underwear to sheets to party favors. Food marketers have ridden the Turtles wave, too. They've created Teenage Mutant Ninja Turtles breakfast cereal, cookies, fruit snacks, frozen pizza, yogurt, pasta, pot pies, and corn snacks.

With the Turtles' love of pizza, a tie-in with a pizza chain was inevitable. Pizza Hut bought into the videocassette release of the original movie. The videotape included a 60-second Pizza Hut commercial, and was packaged with more than $20 in Pizza Hut coupons. Ironically, the movie itself includes a lengthy product placement starring a Domino's Pizza delivery boy. The placement was part of a marketing deal between the movie's producers and Domino's.

Food marketers love tie-ins with cartoons, movies, and video games. The tie-ins bring their products instant recognizability and credibility courtesy of the licensed characters. Just buy the rights to the TMNT name, call your cereal Teenage Mutant Ninja Turtles cereal, and you immediately have millions of children demanding your product. It doesn't matter if the cereal is healthful or not, as long as you slap the magic name on it. Or if you're a fast-food chain, buy the rights to produce action figures based on a popular movie. You'll have millions of kids begging their parents to take them to your outlets.

Movie Madness

Food marketers particularly like tie-ins with movies. In recent years, Ralston Purina has cranked out a flurry of breakfast cereals based on blockbuster movies. In addition to Teenage Mutant Ninja Turtles cereal, other movie tie-ins include Batman Returns, Prince of Thieves cereal and Bill & Ted's Excellent cereal. Earlier, Ralston produced Gremlins, Ghostbusters, Batman, and Jetsons cereals. For the Jetsons cereal, Ralston reportedly spent $10 million on marketing.[16] Other cereal companies haven't been as aggressive as Ralston Purina, although General Mills produced an E.T. cereal and Kellogg rolled out a C-3PO cereal based on *Star Wars*.

Most such cereals exist only as long as the movie is hot. "Generally, a licensed product has a life span of nine months to a year," a Ralston spokesman told *Adweek's Marketing Week*.[17] Ralston has been lucky with some of its cereals, though. The Turtles, for example, seem destined to live for years in movies, TV cartoons, and licensed products.

The short life span of cereals tied into movies doesn't bother food companies, since cranking out a new cereal is relatively easy and cheap. Just mix lots of marshmallows and sugar with a little bit of grain and *voilà!* you've got the perfect tie-in cereal. (Ralston Purina's Ghostbuster II cereal, for example, was about 63 percent sugar.) The box's design is far more important than what's actually inside the box.

The fast-food chains march in lock step with the cereal companies, signing licensing deals with virtually all hot, child-oriented films. Usually, the chains plaster pictures of movie characters on their packaging and cups, and they frequently offer figurines based on the characters. In the past few years, McDonald's has signed licensing deals with such movies as *Jurassic Park, Wayne's World II, Batman Returns, Dick Tracy, Who Framed Roger Rabbit?* and *The Little Mermaid*.

Taco Bell tied into *Free Willy* and *Batman*, Pizza Hut offered sunglasses from *Back to the Future II*, Burger King ran promotions based on *Alvin and the Chipmunks* and *Last Action Hero*, and Wendy's did a promotion with *The Jetsons: The Movie*. Wendy's also handed out six million plastic figurines based on characters in the movie, *All Dogs Go to Heaven*.[18]

Hardee's pushed the outer limits with its promotion for *Ghostbusters II*. Besides offering four different Ghostblaster soundmakers at $1.79 each, the burger chain introduced a special version of its sundae. The topping was bubble-gum-flavored green sauce, which the company said was "reminiscent of the gooey remains from Slimer, a Ghostbuster ghost-lore hero."[19] Yum.

Cartoons

Food marketers love tie-ins with TV cartoons almost as much as those with movies. In recent years, Fred Flintstone and Barney Rubble have pushed Cocoa Pebbles, Fruity Pebbles, Dino Pebbles, John Morell hot dogs, Fruit Juice Fizz, Yabba-Dabba-Doo fruit drink, and Flintstones Push-Up Sherbet Treats;[20] Garfield has promoted PizzOs and Garfield and Friends Fruit Snacks; the Tiny Toon Adventures cast has pitched Tiny Toon Adventures cereal; Bart Simpson has plugged Butterfinger Ice Cream Bars; Snoopy has pushed Snoopy's Choice frozen dinners for kids; and Chip 'n Dale have plugged Chip 'n Dale frozen fudge bars, to name just a few.

Some food marketers are turning to classic cartoon characters like Bugs Bunny. "Classic characters are already proven and definitely safe from backlash," Joni Wilson, product manager for Looney Tunes Meals, told *Adweek's Marketing Week.* "Moms may find the newer characters irritating, but they grew up with Bugs Bunny."[21]

Even the Muppets, stars of public television's *Sesame Street* and their own TV show and movies, succcumbed to commercial temptation. In 1988, Post introduced Croonchy Stars, a cereal "live from the Muppet test kitchens," according to the box. Commercials showed a Muppets character named Swedish Chef making the cereal. Muppets creator Jim Henson developed the cereal's concept.[22]

Finally, there's our personal favorite: Porky Pig plugging Ruffles potato chips. What better pitchman for a high-fat, high-calorie food than a pig?

Video Games

Kids' fascination with video games also has caught food marketers' attention. In 1983, General Mills rolled out Pac-Man cereal, which it introduced with a reported $20 million advertising and promotion budget. A top General Mills executive told *Business Week* why the company licensed the Pac-Man name: "By bringing out a cereal based on Pac-Man, we are not faced with the long, arduous, and expensive task of marketing a brand-new name and identity."[23]

In the late eighties, Ralston Purina rolled out the Nintendo Cereal System, surely one of the strangest cereals ever created. Each box contained two different bags of cereal. One bag had citrus-flavored pieces shaped like the Mario Brothers, while the second held berry-flavored pieces shaped like Zelda. When Ralston launched the cereal, the Mario Brothers and Zelda were characters in Nintendo's two top-selling games.

The Super Mario Brothers game then begat the *Captain N & Super Mario Brothers III* cartoon. And somewhere along the way, Super Mario Bros 3. Assorted Real Fruit Snacks appeared on grocery shelves. As with so many of these creations, it's hard to straighten out which came first: the toy, the cartoon, or the licensed kids' food.

The biggest problem with tie-ins involving food is that they distract kids from the food itself. Kids learn to choose a food because they like the characters on the box, instead of because the food itself is good. Children will choose Batman cereal because they like the movie and comic-book super-hero. The cereal's quality will likely play little or no role in their choice.

To make matters worse, tie-in foods are often the least healthful foods on the market. They're frequently high in sugar, and many are high in fat or sodium as well. Yet if you want to keep your child away from these unhealthy foods, you must fight powerful marketing forces. If your child is obsessed with the Teenage Mutant Ninja Turtles, your refusal to buy Turtles cereal on nutritional grounds can provoke a real battle. Why can't a company produce a low-sugar, high-fiber cereal and plaster a toy or movie's name on the front?

Finally, licensing means paying royalties—typically 5 to 10 percent—to toy companies and movie producers. That means higher prices for consumers.

Product Placements in Movies

It used to be that before the main feature started, movie theaters treated viewers to newsreels, cartoons, or other shorts. Today, though, some theaters have replaced shorts with a stream of lavishly produced commercials. Many of the commercials are designed to look like movie previews, with the sponsor's identity revealed only at the end. That's bad enough. Kids—and adults—shouldn't have to pay good money for the privilege of being a captive audience for commercials.

Even worse is including commercials in the movies themselves. Yet that's exactly what moviemakers are doing more and more frequently. So-called "product placement" produces big bucks and great promotional deals for Hollywood producers. *The Wall Street Journal* estimated that Hollywood collected more than $50 million in product placement fees in 1990. That's more than triple the amount collected just four years earlier, the newspaper said.[24]

If a movie character sips from a Coke can, you can bet it's no accident. In all likelihood, Coke paid a large fee—or offered a generous promotional deal—to get its product shown in the movie. Consumers Union reports that fees can range from

$10,000 to as high as $1,000,000.[25] The fee rises with the prominence of the product's "role" in the movie. For one of its movies, the Walt Disney Company offered to show a brand-name product for $20,000, to mention the product's name while showing it for $40,000, and to have an actor use or hold the product for $60,000.[26]

Food companies got on the product-placement bandwagon after *E.T.* In the 1982 movie—seen by millions of children—the lovable alien gobbled down Reese's Pieces. Within three months after the movie's release, sales of Reese's Pieces soared 66 percent.[27] The movie brought more attention to the candy's name—and in a more alluring way—than any traditional advertising campaign could possibly dream of doing.

Since then, Domino's Pizza and Burger King appeared in *Teenage Mutant Ninja Turtles,* Hardee's and Coca-Cola appeared in *Days of Thunder,* Burger King and Coors beer showed up in *Gremlins,* and Pizza Hut was featured in *Back to the Future II,* to name just a few roles.[28]

In 1990, five of the six top-grossing films had a total of 148 references to brand-name products, according to the Center for the Study of Commercialism. One of these, *Home Alone,* the third-highest-grossing movie of 1990, had references to 31 brand names. Food products shown or mentioned included Pepsi, Reddi Wip whipped cream, Junior Mints candy, Crunch Tators snack food, Kraft marshmallows, Skittles candy, Freshen Up gum, Chiclets gum, Cheez Curls, Tropicana orange juice, Kraft Macaroni & Cheese, and Tic Tac breath mints.[29]

Among food companies, PepsiCo is probably the most aggressive in buying movie roles for its products. Pepsi products have appeared in such films as *Ferris Bueller's Day Off, Stand and Deliver, Teenage Mutant Ninja Turtles, Lean on Me, Cocoon: The Return, Flashdance, Big, Back to the Future II, Total Recall, Ghost,* and *Home Alone.*[30]

Frequently, fast-food chains whose products appear in movies unleash major promotions tied to the films. Burger King tied the beginning of its Kids Club to *Teenage Mutant Ninja Turtles,* McDonald's ran a big *Dick Tracy* contest, and Pizza Hut sold futuristic sunglasses based on *Back to the Future.*

The award for most blatant out-and-out hucksterism goes to *Mac and Me.* The 1988 Orion movie masqueraded as a cheap rip-off of *E.T.* It's about a boy who befriends an alien, Mac, who has been separated from its family. Actually, it was little more than a 99-minute commercial for McDonald's, Coca-Cola, and Sears. It's probably no accident that the three companies featured in the movie have strong connections to each other. McDonald's sells Coke products exclusively, and Sears sells the McKids line of clothing.

Numerous companies have sprung up to broker deals for firms that want to place their products in movies. In pitches to potential clients, the companies make no effort to hide what they do. "Brand name products can't sing . . . they can't dance . . . nor can they act," Silver Screen Placements Inc. wrote to potential clients. "But, they *do* receive almost as much attention as their human counterparts. Imagine the impact of *your* customers seeing *their* favorite star using *your* product in a feature film or TV show. Both YOUR COMPANY'S NAME AND PRODUCT thereby become an integral part of the show, conveying both subliminal messages and implied endorsements."[31]

Another company, Associated Film Productions, claims to have placed brand-name products in nearly 600 major films during its first five years in business. "AFP carefully controls the appearance of the client's product in films," wrote President Robert Kovoloff in a letter to prospective clients. "In most cases, it is the stars who will use the product—always in a positive and memorable manner. Great care is taken to prevent a product from being used by villains or in a disparaging way."

Kovoloff boasted of his firm's close ties to Hollywood producers. "Producers and directors frequently ask AFP to recommend ways in which brand-name products can be creatively used to enhance a scene," he wrote. "This has led to many beneficial exposures of products in specially devised scenes that have great brand-name impact."[32]

A coalition of consumer groups, led by the Center for the Study of Commercialism, blasted product placements in a petition filed in 1991 with the Federal Trade Commission. "Product placements are designed with the intent to deceive and exploit unsuspecting consumers . . . ," the groups said. "Such intentional deception contravenes public policy because it is unethical and unfair to consumers. . . ."[33]

The groups asked the FTC to require studios to run notices at the beginning of movies that feature brand-name products. The notice would say: "The motion picture you are about to see contains advertisements for the following products, paid for by the following companies . . ." The consumer groups realized that such notices would be meaningless to children, so they asked the FTC to ban paid product placements in movies directed at children.

Representative Ron Wyden (D-Ore.), chairman of the House Subcommittee on Regulation, Business Opportunities, and Energy, supported the groups' petition. "I was shocked to learn that product manufacturers pay thousands of dollars to advertise through product placement to unsuspecting audiences," he wrote in a letter to the FTC. In late 1992, however, the FTC denied the petition.

While all product placements are deceptive, those for foods have special potential to harm children. That's because almost invariably, the foods placed in movies are unhealthful. In *Mac and Me* a child sees the cute alien living on just Coke and Skittles. Coke even stars as a miracle drink that revives dying aliens. Those are powerful messages. They have great potential to confuse young children whose parents are encouraging them to develop healthy eating habits.

Premiums

It's a hot summer afternoon as the long-suffering parent drives a minivan full of boisterous kids home from the pool. They're hungry. Where to eat?

Fast food is the obvious choice. Eighty percent of all restaurant meals eaten by kids under 18 are at fast-food restaurants, according to the National Restaurant Association.[34] But how to choose among the joints that line streets in virtually every American city?

The debate raging in the backseat over where to eat isn't likely to center on which restaurant has the most nutritious offerings. Nor are the kids likely to wrangle over which place has the most efficient service, the cleanest bathrooms, or even the tastiest food.

Instead, the debate likely concerns one issue: Who's giving away the best toy? Will it be California Raisins Claymation figures at Hardee's, car-shaped erasers at KFC, ALF magnets at Burger King, a Potato Head Kid at Wendy's, Matchbox cars at Rax, or a Funny Fry Friend at McDonald's? Since many of these toys come in sets ("Collect all four!"), the decision can get pretty complicated—and expensive.

The next day, the long-suffering parent takes a couple of his or her young children to the grocery store. The kids run ahead to the cereal aisle, where the store has thoughtfully placed kids' cereals on the lower shelves. Some kids choose the same cereal every time, others want a cereal tied in to a movie or cartoon, and others pick one because they like its commercials. Lots of children, though, race from box to box looking for the best premium. In fact, when researchers from Michigan State University asked mothers what reasons their 3- to 11-year-old children gave when requesting a specific cereal, just over 80 percent said the child wanted the premium inside the box. Mothers listed this motive far more often than any other.[35]

In another study, the MSU researchers watched parents and their children in the supermarket cereal aisle. Nearly half the children appeared to consider the premium when choosing a cereal, according to the researchers. When parents expressed reluctance to buy a cereal for a premium, the parent and child typically fought in the supermarket.[36]

Premiums with kids' foods are nothing new. In 1933, a kid could get a Babe Ruth movie book by sending Wheaties one box top. But today, premiums are playing an increasingly critical role in food marketing.

"To a kid, a hamburger is a hamburger is a hamburger, so you have to have a more attractive premium," Wendy's spokesman Denny Lynch told *The Wall Street Journal*. "We can't outmaneuver McDonald's on Saturday morning TV, but we can beat them on the quality of premiums."[37]

This one-upmanship with premiums can get expensive. Gone are the days when a penny piece of plastic molded into a tiny ship, car, or ring would satisfy a child. Today, some fast-food chains are handing out premiums that wholesale for anywhere from a quarter to 90 cents.[38] Of course, the chains pass along those costs through higher prices.

Increasingly, fast-food chains are offering upscale premiums and charging separately for them. Burger King offered five different *Simpsons* toys for $3.49 each, Hardee's charged $1.79 each for four different Ghostblaster soundmakers, Pizza Hut charged $1.99 for its *Back to the Future* sunglasses, and Wendy's sold a series of plush leopards, tigers, pandas, and koalas for $2.19 each. For a parent, paying a few bucks for a premium on top of the meal adds significantly to the cost of eating fast food.

Costs really mount if a child insists on returning each week to collect the next toy in the set.

For fast-food restaurants, the whole point of premiums is to hook children initially and then keep them coming back. That's why they offer so many premiums in sets that require children to return each week to collect the next toy.

The worst thing about premiums, though, is that they encourage kids to choose foods based on the toys that come with them, instead of choosing a food based on the taste and nutritional value. Meals simply become opportunities to collect more toys.

Tie-ins With Toys and Clothes

If you walk down the play-food aisle of a major toy store today, you may do a double take. Have you somehow taken a wrong turn and ended up on a fast-food strip? On one side are McDonald's Happy Meals, Burger King Whoppers, and banana splits from Baskin-Robbins. On the other are Dunkin' Donuts, Swanson TV dinners, and Pepsi bottles. Food marketers have taken over the aisle as they try to get you to pay good money for "toys" that do little more than promote their products.

Most commonly, toy companies make plastic imitations of heavily advertised foods. Some wags might argue that the imitation food and the real food are hard to tell apart, since they're both plastic. Toy companies even add scents to some of the plastic foods, like the Baskin-Robbins banana splits, to increase the realism.

For kids who want to make fast food from clay, Play-Doh offers Burger King and Pizza Hut playsets. And if children want to cook real fast food, they can use the Domino's Pizza oven to make mini pizzas from mixes.

McDonald's is the most aggressive company in plastering its name on kids' toys and clothes. It has teamed up with Fisher-Price to churn out a never-ending stream of plastic toys featuring the golden arches.

By far the biggest toy is a child-size plastic McDonald's Restaurant. It has everything: a grill and fryer, a walk-up counter and cash register, and a drive-through window. It also comes with plastic hamburgers, pickles, fries, a fry scoop, a spatula, trays, and coins, and retails for about $90.

If the McDonald's Restaurant is a little pricey, you can choose between the McDonald's Soda Fountain and the McDonald's Cooking Center with pretend fry warmer, fryer, and hamburger grill (both about $30). Finally, there are the McDonald's restaurant that Mattel created for Barbie and Fisher-Price's Little People McDonald's Restaurant. The Fisher-Price restaurant comes with a miniature playground and Ronald McDonald, Hamburglar, and Little People figures.

While playing with all these toys, a child needs a McDonald's Crew Uniform (about $10). The truly well-dressed child, though, needs a whole wardrobe of McKids clothes from Sears—sweaters, pants, skirts, shorts, "activewear," "nightwear," jeans, and shoes, all emblazoned with the McDonald's arches. Sears refuses to release sales figures for the McKids line. However, an *Adweek* columnist estimated that Sears could rake in $200 million to $300 million annually from McKids.[39]

Burger King hasn't surrendered the toy stores to McDonald's. Mattel, which makes a McDonald's restaurant for Barbie, also produces a Burger King restaurant for Barbie's cousin, Jazzie. The restaurant set, liberally splashed with Burger King's name and logo, retails for about $30. In the picture on the box, Jazzie and other dolls are holding tiny plastic Burger King sandwiches or trays. If you peer very carefully, you can make out the box's small type: "Dolls cannot hold accessories as shown."

Plastic hamburgers, fast-food restaurants for Barbie, and all the other food-related toys covered with corporate logos encourage kids' love affairs with unhealthful foods. If a child makes a Burger King Whopper with his Play-Doh set, how many minutes pass until he demands that his parents take him to Burger King for the real thing? Toys like that also get commercial messages into a child's playroom, a place that—ideally—should be free of commercial pressures.

Marketers' use of brand-name food toys, kids clubs, tie-ins with movies and TV shows, product placements in films, and premiums continues to grow. However, those efforts pale in comparison to companies' favorite method for hooking kids: television commercials. That's where we turn next.

CHAPTER 7

Television, the Sneaky Salesmachine

Imagine this scene: a door-to-door salesman raps on your door. When you open it, he says: "Good morning. I'd like to beguile your children and lure them into bad habits that will harm their health. Please leave the room so I can speak to them directly without your interference."

Would you welcome this salesman into your home? Of course not—you'd slam the door and call the police instead. Yet a slick version of this salesman visits virtually every home in America on a daily basis. He's welcomed into millions of living rooms, family rooms, and even children's bedrooms.

This slick salesman is television, the electronic descendant of the door-to-door huckster. When it comes to bewitching children, television commercials are far more effective than any human salesperson ever was. Marketers of children's products love TV because commercials bypass parents and directly grab the target audience: kids. Then many of the kids ask their parents to buy whatever they saw advertised. If the kids' first request doesn't succeed, the commercials remind them to keep asking again and again. Sooner or later, even the most conscientious parent is likely to give in—at least some of the time.

Back in the 1970s, there was a brief, shining moment when

it looked as if the federal government might ban all television advertising to young children. Then—as now—a ban was justified by compelling evidence showing that TV commercials were simply unfair. They're particularly unfair to young children, who often can't separate commercials from programs and don't understand that commercials are trying to sell them something.

Yet today, some 15 years after a ban appeared possible, commercials targeting kids jam the airwaves. Many of them push foods—almost always presweetened breakfast cereals, soft drinks, candy bars, fast-food meals, and other foods that are high in sugar, fat, or salt. While government watchdogs sleep comfortably, lots of the food commercials violate the letter or spirit of federal regulations or industry guidelines designed to ensure that TV commercials are fair to children.

How did we get from a possible ban on commercials aimed at children to today's wide-open marketplace? The tale is a disheartening one. Before we begin it, though, we must first explore the nature of TV advertising to children.

What TV Tells Kids About Food

The colors and moving images on television attract children virtually from birth. Commercials, with their fast-moving pictures, bright colors, and snappy music, are especially alluring. In one study, 6-month-old infants got so interested in television that they cried when researchers turned off the sound but left on the picture.[1]

Children develop the television habit early. By ages 2 to 5, the average child watches nearly four hours of television daily, according to the A.C. Nielsen Company. By ages 6 to 11, when children have begun school, their viewing drops slightly to about three and one-half hours daily. And in the teen years, it drops further to just over three hours per day.[2]

Children spend more time watching TV than doing anything else except sleeping, according to University of Michigan professor Bruce Watkins. The Consumers Union, publisher of *Consumer Reports* magazine, estimates that the average child potentially sees between 30,000 and 40,000 commercials annually.[3] Of course, no one knows how channel switching, zapping, or going to the bathroom affects the number of commercials that children actually watch.

The average child sees about 350,000 to 400,000 TV commercials by the time he or she graduates from high school. Keep in mind that is just the average. Heavy TV viewers could easily see half a million commercials or even more by graduation.

The heaviest TV viewers frequently come from low-income families. Figures from Nielsen, the TV-research firm, show that low-income children ages 2 to 11 watch an average of 33 hours per week. That compares to 22 hours weekly for their middle-income peers and 19 hours for high-income children.[4] Ironically, it's the children from poor families who see the most advertising messages urging them to spend lots of money.

Whether rich or poor, children learn a tremendous amount about the world from watching both television programs and commercials. Television—like parents, schools, and religious institutions—"imparts many messages to children about society, its values, and its expectations," Professor Watkins said.[5] Food commercials are part of this socialization process. A National Science Foundation report cited research indicating "that a child's developing sense of what our culture deems fit to eat is influenced by the foods that he or she sees in television commercials."[6]

Unfortunately, a child watching TV commercials gets a truly perverted view of what society thinks is best to eat. Nearly all the food commercials shown during children's programs push

Non-Nutritious Messages

In a pre-Christmas survey undertaken in 1992, CSPI found that food commercials comprised 29 percent of the 362 commercials and public service messages aired on Saturday morning.* (The majority of commercials were—surprise, surprise—for toys.) There was only one PSA, promoting good nutrition; it emphasized eating fresh vegetables. There wasn't a single word to discourage kids from eating fatty or sugary foods.

FOOD	NUMBER	PERCENTAGE
Breakfast cereals	52	49%
Fast food	30	28%
Candy	11	10%
Drinks/chocolate syrup	8	7%
Milk	3	3%
Cookies	1	1%
Nutrition public service announcement	1	1%

*Survey by Center for Science in the Public Interest, Nov., 1992, commercials on 18.5 hours of Saturday-morning broadcasts on ABC, CBS, Fox, and Nickelodeon.

foods high in sugar, fat, or salt, according to a study commissioned by the Council of Better Business Bureaus. Commercials for sugary cereals, snacks, drinks, and fast food account for almost half of all commercials on kids' shows. Commercials for healthy foods such as milk, fruit, and vegetables rarely appear. They make up less than 3 percent of all commercials during kids' programs.[7]

The Center for Science in the Public Interest (CSPI) found similar patterns in February 1991 when it analyzed Saturday-morning commercials on ABC, NBC, CBS, Fox, and Nickelodeon. CSPI found that nearly two-thirds of the commercials pushed food. And nine out of ten food commercials promoted candy bars, sugary cereals, snack foods, salty canned foods, fast food, and chips.

Of the 222 food commercials broadcast during 20 hours of programming, only 8 were for reasonably healthy products. Those included low-sugar cereals, frozen entrées, and milk. A "good breakfast" commercial sponsored by Kellogg was the sole commercial or public service announcement (PSA) that plugged eating fresh, unprocessed food. Clearly, a single message advocating a good breakfast cannot compete with the flood of commercials for nutritionally flawed foods. For PSAs to be effective, they must use the same high production standards as commercials and must run frequently. Major advertisers—such as General Mills, which paid its chief executive, H. Brewster Atwater, Jr., $8 million in 1991[8]—couldn't find the funds to sponsor a single nutrition message.

The advertising situation may be getting worse than ever, according to researchers at the pediatrics department of Columbia University. When they compared the kinds of ads broadcast in 1989 to those broadcast in 1993, they found that commercials for high-fat foods (mostly fast foods) jumped from 16 percent to 41 percent of all food advertising. Apparently, the guidelines encouraging lower-fat diets for children issued in 1991 by the National Cholesterol Education Program did not temper the fast-food industry's efforts to tempt kids.[9]

Compounding the problem is the fact that most kids, particularly those below age 10 or so, actually like TV commercials. "If a station were to program non-stop commercials for children, it's quite possible they could attract a sizable audience," said Dale Kunkel, an assistant professor of communications at the University of California–Santa Barbara who has written widely about kids and TV. "Kids like commercials a lot."

That is not surprising, considering the huge sums of money

that food companies spend to design, produce, and air TV commercials aimed at attracting them. Fast-food, soft-drink, and snack-food companies spend an average of a quarter-million dollars to create a single TV spot.[10] In 1992, McDonald's alone spent $388 million to air TV commercials, Coca-Cola spent $202 million, and General Mills spent $407 million.[11] Many of those companies' commercials are pitched at children and teenagers.

If kids love TV commercials and companies happily spend millions airing them, what's the beef? Why should the government regulate television advertising to children?

There are two reasons. First, advertising to young children is inherently unfair and deceptive. Unfair and deceptive commercials are particularly abhorrent when they involve food because they can dramatically affect children's lifelong eating habits and health. The second reason is that TV stations are licensed to use the airwaves in the public interest. The government shouldn't let them get away with harming the very public that owns those airwaves.

TV's Tricky Tactics

The deception in commercials aimed at kids takes many forms. For starters, many children below the age of 5 cannot consistently tell the difference between commercials and programs. That leaves them no defenses against commercial messages, no ability to raise red flags that say, "Hey, I should watch this commercial differently from how I watch the program."

Yet even those young children who can separate commercials from programs still don't understand a commercial's selling intent until they're at least age 7 or 8. And even once they do understand the nature of commercials, they don't recognize that

The Power of Public Action

ONLY PROMPT ACTION by children's advocates stopped Chester Cheetah, the cartoon character who appears in commercials for Frito-Lay's Chee-tos snack, from starring in his own TV show.

The Fox Broadcasting Company was developing an animated program called *Yo! It's Chester Cheetah!* for possible inclusion in its Saturday-morning schedule in fall 1992. Fox officials claimed they had only the purest motives in using a commercial pitch-animal in a TV program aimed at kids.

"Believe me, the fact that [this character] was attached to Frito-Lay was irrelevant," Margaret Loesch, president of the Fox Children's Network, told *Inside Media* in March 1992. "We decided we would not run Chee-tos commercials adjacent to the show, or perhaps not on Saturday mornings at all. We thought this was one of the best characters since Bugs Bunny."

Children's advocates disagreed, seeing the show as a blatant attempt to air a half-hour commercial in the guise of a children's program. In March 1992, Action for Children's Television, the Center for Science in the Public Interest, and five other groups petitioned the FCC to block the show. The groups said the program would be "inherently deceptive," because it would confuse children about the difference between programs and commercials.

Less than two weeks after the groups filed their petition, Fox dropped the show. Fox officials claimed that problems in negotiating for use of the character—not the petition—doomed the program. But the timing does seem curious, doesn't it?

advertisers may exaggerate their claims and omit important facts about the product. Many studies dating back nearly two decades have conclusively proven that point.[12]

If kids don't understand the selling intent of commercials, they trust them just as much as programs. When Fred Flintstone appears in a Cocoa Pebbles commercial and tells them the cereal tastes good and is nutritious, kids believe him. That's partly because they see him all the time in cartoons they love. If they don't understand the intent of commercials, how are children to know that Fred plays a far different role in the Cocoa Pebbles commercial than he does in the cartoon?

That misplaced trust revealed itself when researchers from Michigan State University showed a Cocoa Pebbles commercial to a group of 4- to 7-year-olds. In the commercial, Fred Flintstone and Barney Rubble said the cereal was "chocolatey enough to make you smile." After watching it, more than half the children said they wanted the cereal because Fred and Barney liked it.[13]

Dale Kunkel is blunt in assessing whether it's fair to advertise to young children. "I don't think it's in the public interest to shoot fish in a barrel, which is what you're doing advertising to children below the age of about 7 to 8 years," he said. He added that 7 to 8 "is a very conservative estimate of the age at which finally it is fair to advertise to children."

As the Cocoa Pebbles commercial illustrates, marketers try to further confuse kids about the difference between programs and commercials by using stars from their favorite cartoons as commercial pitchmen. "For the young child, it's harder to appreciate that there are programs and there are commercials when the same characters appear in both on a regular basis," Kunkel said.

To blur the line even further, television stations sometimes run commercials with a cartoon character back-to-back with programs starring the same character. For example, between shows during one afternoon of cartoons on the Fox station in Washington, D.C., Barney Rubble and Fred Flintstone appeared in a commercial for Cocoa Pebbles cereal. Less than a minute after the commercial ended, the opening theme for *The Flintstones* cartoon started.[14] A young child could easily have had difficulty separating the commercial from the program.

That potential for confusion is why in 1974 the Federal Communications Commission banned the practice of "host selling." In a report, the FCC said "basic fairness requires that . . . a clear separation be maintained between the program content and the commercial message"[15] to help children distinguish between them.

Some TV stations, like the one in Washington, blithely ignore the FCC's ban on host selling. There's little chance they'll be caught, and even if caught it's unlikely they'll suffer any penalty worse than a slap on the wrist.

To add to the confusion, some broadcasters leave out separation devices between programs and commercials. In a separator, a character typically says: "We'll be right back after these messages." That's a subtle signal to kids that a commercial is next. At the end of the commercial, a character usually says: "Now, back to our program." The separators are supposed to help kids differentiate programs from commercials.

Although the FCC requires these separators, broadcasters frequently "forget" to insert them. Fifteen percent of commercial breaks on kids' programs lack one or both separators, according to a study Kunkel performed for the Better Business Bureau. Independent stations violate the requirement most often. They leave out separators in one of every four commercial breaks.[16]

Stations keep violating the rules because the FCC doesn't actively enforce them, Kunkel said. The FCC only acts when someone files a complaint against a station.

Another favorite tactic of advertisers is to include confusing or downright misleading nutrition information. Charles Atkin, a Michigan State University professor who did pioneering research on children and television in the 1970s, found that children readily believe nutrition claims (for example, "high in vitamin C" or "good for you") in commercials. "Although children are skeptical about assertions in commercials for familiar toys, they readily accept technical claims of a medical or nutritional nature," Atkin wrote. "Heavy viewers of commercials are more likely to believe commercials than are light viewers."[17]

Kids, particularly those who watch lots of TV, even believe implied nutrition claims. For example, a group of 4- to 7-year-olds watched a commercial where a circus strongman lifted a playhouse after eating a cereal. Almost two-thirds of the children thought eating the cereal would make them stronger.[18]

Other studies have found that heavy TV viewers have the poorest nutrition knowledge. In one study, kids who watched lots of TV were twice as likely as light viewers to believe that sugared cereals and candy are highly nutritious.[19] In another, seven out of ten kids thought McDonald's food was more nutritious than what their parents served at home.[20] (We hope those kids were wrong!)

Why are kids so confused by nutrition claims in food commercials? Mainly because marketers employ clever tricks. Consider cereal commercials, which may have the most confusing nutrition claims of any food ads. Their poor quality is particularly disturbing because cereal is the food most heavily advertised to children. Between one-fifth[21] and one-third[22] of all TV commercials during children's programs push cereals. This means that children who watch 30,000 commercials in a year see between 6,000 and 10,000 cereal commercials.

The typical cereal commercial is a visual and audio feast, with animated characters, bouncy music, and fast action. Amidst all the frenzy, it's easy to miss the nutrition information. But it's there. It consists of an audio "disclaimer" and a quick picture of a breakfast table.

Disclaimers vary slightly. Typically, an announcer or character in the commercial says the cereal is "part of a complete breakfast," "part of a nutritious breakfast," or "part of a balanced breakfast." While someone reads the phrase, a breakfast table flashes on the screen for a few seconds. Breakfast tables shown in various commercials are amazingly similar. The cereal appears front and center, almost invariably accompanied by milk, orange juice, and toast. Among commercials for 18 different kids' cereals, 11 showed this breakfast spread. The others added a muffin or some fruit.

Advertisers include the audio disclaimers and breakfast pictures for two reasons: to comply with industry guidelines and so they can claim that their commercials include "nutrition information." The industry guidelines were developed by the Children's Advertising Review Unit (CARU) of the Council of Better Business Bureaus. The advertising industry created the CARU to monitor advertising practices.

The guidelines say commercials should show foods in ways that "encourage sound usage of the product with a view toward healthy development of the child and the development of good nutritional practices. Advertisements representing mealtime in the home should clearly and adequately depict the role of the product within the framework of a balanced diet."[23]

The guidelines are nice. In theory, they make commercials more informative. But in practice, they may actually lead to confusion and deception. Disclaimers are the biggest culprits. What do they actually tell children? "Usually, they don't tell them anything," said Robert Liebert, who teaches psychology at the State University of New York at Stony Brook and has studied kids and TV since the 1960s. Disclaimers are too short to help much and often occur in a context that contradicts them, Liebert said.

One of the reasons disclaimers are uninformative is that they use language kids can't understand. "Though nominally they are in English, practically speaking they are in a foreign language to the child," Liebert said. What exactly does "part of a complete breakfast" mean to a child? Does it mean the breakfast isn't complete without the heavily sugared cereal?

Liebert particularly objects to advertisers who use the phrase "part of a nutritious breakfast." He said this phrase is "the most misleading because that's a very complicated idea for a child to understand. It's very, very easy for the child to believe that the overwhelming nutritional contribution is made by the cereal, instead of by the other things that are for a mere moment pictured on the breakfast table as part of the commercial."

Showing the cereal on the breakfast table with other foods also doesn't increase kids' nutritional understanding. Advertisers show the table because the CARU guidelines require that a food be shown "within the framework of a balanced diet." The theory is that if kids see the foods together, they'll realize they need to eat all of them to get a "complete" breakfast.

Unfortunately, several studies have found that most kids do not notice the other foods that appear with the cereal. In one study using 4- to 7-year-olds, Atkin and a colleague at Michigan State University showed the children a cereal commercial. They then asked the kids to recall what foods appeared on the breakfast table with the cereal. Two-thirds couldn't remember a single food.[24]

Food Commercials That Sell Fun

Besides trying their darnedest to confuse kids, food advertisers also work hard to attract them with something other than the food itself. Most commonly, they tout premiums in their commercials.

Fast-food commercials feature premiums the most. Premiums appear in about one-third of fast-food commercials aired during kids' shows, according to a study commissioned by the CARU.[25] Because premiums can increase a child's desire for a product, the CARU urges advertisers to pay "special attention" when advertising premiums "to guard against exploiting children's immaturity."[26] Yet about one in six commercials touting premiums violates the standards, according to the CARU.[27]

Most frequently, the commercials violate a prohibition against focusing more on the premium than the product. The CARU guideline states: "If product advertising contains a premium message, care should be taken that the child's attention is focused primarily on the product. The premium message should be clearly secondary."

You don't have to watch much children's TV to spot food commercials where the premium plays the starring role. For example, a 30-second Burger King spot showed:

- Animated Kids Club leaders preparing a meal: 12 seconds.
- A child playing with the premium, a Captain Planet Star Cruiser: 11 seconds.
- Four Star Cruisers, a drink cup, and a food bag together on a table, with the premiums prominently in front: 4 seconds.
- A plug for the Kids Club: 3 seconds.

Obviously, the premium was more prominent than the food. But the CARU has no power to enforce its guidelines. It can ask companies to pull specific commercials, but it can't force them to do so.

In this virtually unregulated marketplace, lots of companies join Burger King in violating the spirit of the CARU premium guideline. For example, a 30-second McDonald's commercial showed Ronald McDonald working with kids in their garden for 15 seconds. It then showed for 15 seconds mini garden tools that McDonald's was giving away as premiums.

Companies have powerful incentives to violate the premium guideline because, as we saw in Chapter 5, premiums strongly influence children's food choices, with kids often choosing a product or restaurant solely because of its premium.

Kids' focus on premiums rises with the amount of television

Milk as Miracle Nutrient

EREAL COMMERCIALS aren't the only ads making dubious nutritional claims. A commercial for milk, the all-American beverage, takes high honors for deception.

It opens with a muscle-bound hunk, dressed in a T-shirt and jeans, sitting in a high school locker room drinking milk. "Milk is sure helping me get stronger," he says. The scene shifts to his first year in high school. He's short and nerdy. Two tough-looking guys, who are at least a few inches taller, push him out of the way in the hall. "Back when I started high school, guys used to push me around just because I was smaller," he says.

Then he explains that he kept drinking milk and working out. The scene shifts back to the present, when he's all muscle. He runs into the same tough-looking guys in the hall. This time he's an inch taller than they are, and he elbows them out of the way. "As you can see, it pays to be big on milk," he says.

The message is that drinking milk helped transform this geek into a Charles Atlas—and in just two short years. The commercial mentions that he worked out, but downplays this factor. Milk comes across as a miracle food, a magic elixir that can solve the problems of adolescence.

Milk does contain many

they watch on Saturday mornings, according to a survey Atkin did of mothers. Seventy percent of kids who watched an hour or less on Saturday mornings requested a cereal because of premiums. That compares with 86 percent of children who watched two hours or more and 90 percent of those who watched three hours or more.[28]

In 1974, the Federal Trade Commission asked advertisers voluntarily to stop mentioning premiums in their TV commercials, contending that featuring premiums in commercials was unfair and harmful to children. The FTC declared that "the

valuable nutrients that help growing bodies, but its powers don't extend to converting wimps into hunks. The commercial clearly violates a Children's Advertising Review Unit (CARU) guideline that bars deception about a product's benefits. "The advertising presentation should not mislead children about perceived benefits from use of the product," the guideline states. "Such benefits may include, but are not limited to, the acquisition of *strength, status,* popularity, *growth,* proficiency, and intelligence" (emphasis added).

Any wimp considering drinking gallons of whole milk also better be aware that the saturated fat in milk can help clog arteries, a process that's often well under way by the teen years. A glass of whole milk has 5 grams of saturated fat—that's one-fourth or more of most youngsters' daily limit. Drinking three glasses of milk over the day would eat up practically all of a child's saturated-fat quota.

Two percent milk isn't much better. Each glass has about 3 grams of saturated fat, and three glasses would supply half of a child's saturated-fat quota. Only 1 percent lowfat milk and skim milk are truly low in fat. The milk commercial doesn't discuss fat at all. Big surprise, huh?

premium's main purpose is to distract the buyer's attention from [the product's] attributes and to motivate purchase not on the merits of the products but in order to obtain the premium."[29] A few years later, though, the FTC dropped its suggested ban on premium advertising.

Many food commercials aimed at kids emphasize fun. Frequently, those commercials show groups of kids having a great time while eating the food. The fun theme is especially big in fast-food commercials, with seven out of ten using this appeal.[30]

A Burger King commercial plugging its Kids Club is a classic example of the genre. The commercial showed a whole group of kids at Burger King doing cartwheels and otherwise whooping it up. The clear implication was that kids who joined the club would become part of a group where they met lots of new friends and had loads of fun.

"The ad was deceptive because it implied that going to Burger King for a child was like going to a club meeting," said Peggy Charren, founder of the now-defunct Action for Children's Television. "The fact is that going to get a hamburger is not like going to a Boy Scout meeting or to a Boys Club or a Girls Club or whatever. It's a restaurant. We felt that kids were being encouraged to go to Burger King for the wrong reasons."

ACT filed a complaint with the Federal Trade Commission, alleging that the commercial was deceptive. But the FTC never formally acted on the complaint. Instead, it kicked the issue to the industry-backed CARU, which was then developing guidelines about kids clubs. In 1991, the CARU issued a guideline that stated: "In advertising to children, care should be taken not to mislead them into thinking they are joining a club when they are merely making a purchase or receiving a premium." The Burger King commercial clearly violates the new guideline.

How Food Commercials Affect Our Kids' Health

As deceptive as food commercials are, they'd be of less concern if they had no impact on kids' food choices or their health. Unfortunately, several studies have found that commercials greatly affect what kids eat. In one study, 5- to 8-year-old children attending summer camp in Canada were split into two groups. Both groups saw a 30-minute cartoon each day. One group saw it with commercials for candies and Kool-Aid. The other group saw the cartoon with commercials for various fruits and yogurt.

After viewing the cartoons and commercials each day, the kids chose snacks. Counselors told them to choose one of two beverages and two of four foods. The beverages were Kool-Aid and orange juice; the foods were usually two candy bars and two fruits.

The commercials strongly affected the kids' food choices. Forty-five percent of those who saw an orange juice commercial chose orange juice. Only 25 percent of the kids who saw the Kool-Aid commercial picked orange juice over Kool-Aid. And of the kids who saw fruit commercials, 36 percent chose fruit as a snack, compared to 25 percent of those who saw candy ads.

Two other researchers, both of whom once worked on children's advertising issues for the Federal Trade Commission, reviewed nine experimental studies of kids and TV commercials and concluded that commercials strongly affect what kids eat. "Exposure to commercials for sugared products leads to greater consumption of sugared products, greater preference for sugared foods—even unadvertised sugared foods—and lower nutrition knowledge," they wrote.[31] The same conclusion undoubtedly applies to commercials for high-fat foods as well.

Consistently, experts have found that kids who watch the most TV have the worst diets and the lowest levels of nutritional knowledge. A researcher at the University of Massachusetts found that as kids' television viewing climbed, so did the likelihood they ate heavily sugared cereals, candy, and snack foods.[32]

Television's influence is most obvious when researchers examine what children ask for at the supermarket. A report by the New York State Assembly said that "children who cannot yet walk or read will recognize a product by its package and reach for it from the shopping cart."[33] How do they recognize the package? They've seen it on TV.

The Case of the Missing Fruit

AS THE COMMERCIAL opens, a young boy sits down to eat Froot Loops with Toucan Sam.

"Hey Toucan, how do you get such a big fruit taste from these little Froot Loops?" asks the boy.

"You mean that mondo, mega-fruit taste?" replies the bird.

"Umm, yeah," says the boy.

"Simple," says the bird. Huge fruits—an orange, a lemon, and cherries—fall from the sky, landing next to them. The fruits are bigger than either the boy or the bird.

"Big fruit!" exclaims the boy.

"Mondo, mega-fruit!" Toucan Sam agrees.

"Yes," chimes in an announcer. "You'll love the humongous orange, gigantic lemon, and mammoth cherry flavors of Kellogg's Froot Loops." Toucan Sam reinforces the message. "Kellogg's Froot Loops," he says. "Big fruit taste from big fruit."

Based on the commercial, a child—or even an adult—could easily think Froot Loops is chock-full of fruit. The label reinforces that impression. It states that a one-ounce serving provides 100 percent of the U.S. Recommended Daily Allowance of vitamin C. That's one of the nutrients found in abundance in most real fruit.

Actually, though, Froot Loops doesn't contain *any* fruit. Near the bottom of the label's ingredient list are the words "natural orange, lemon, and cherry and other natural *flavorings.*" Where does all the vitamin C come from? Kellogg's dumps it in as an additive.

What Froot Loop *does* contain is a lot of sugar. It's 46 percent sugar—13 grams (or 3¼ teaspoons) in a one-ounce serving.

Donna Thede, Kellogg's publicity manager, said the fruit falling from the sky in the commercial is designed to show "the variety of flavors included in the cereal. We have a team of Ph.D. nutritionists and registered dietitians and attorneys who review all our commercials and approve them, and we do not feel we put out deceptive advertising."

Nonetheless, researchers have found that commercials such as the Froot Loops spot do trick kids into thinking there's real fruit in the product. In one study at the University of Kansas, grade-school children who saw commercials for foods with artificial fruit flavorings frequently believed the foods contained real fruit.

Cereal boxes can be just as deceptive as TV commercials. The box for Trix, made by General Mills, contains phrases like "fruity frosted corn puffs," "more fruit flavor," "real grape juice," and "good source of vitamin C." For good measure, it also includes a picture of an orange, a lime, a lemon, and grapes.

The only fruit in Trix is a tiny quantity of grape juice concentrate. The vitamin C is added rather than natural.

Even more deceptive are the so-called "fruit snacks" that have flooded the market recently. They contain virtually no fruit. "A serving of most of the major brands has the equivalent of one and a half grapes or one-seventeenth of an orange," Bonnie F. Liebman, nutrition director at the Center for Science in the Public Interest,

said. "Overall, these are Gummi Bears. They are just like candy."

"Don't be deceived when you see fruit listed first on the ingredient label," she added. "Fruit just weighs a lot because it's 90 percent water." Labels list ingredients by weight, so fruit often tops the list.

To determine the fruit content, check how much vitamin C the fruit snack contains. Almost invariably, fruit snacks contain less than 2 percent of the U.S. RDA of vitamin C, which means you're probably not getting much fruit. Likewise, if the snack contains lots of vitamin C, check the ingredient list for ascorbic acid (vitamin C). If it's listed, the manufacturer has dumped in vitamin C as an additive.

One study, conducted by researchers at Columbia University's Teachers College, found that the more commercial television preschoolers watched, the more foods they asked for when shopping with their parents.

What did the kids request most? Cereals and candy, which not coincidentally are two of the foods most heavily advertised to children. Among children who requested cereal, nearly seven out of ten asked for a sugared cereal. Nearly 10 percent of the kids requested specific brand names, usually ones that were advertised heavily on TV. The researchers acknowledged they couldn't prove a cause-and-effect relationship between television viewing and purchase demands. Still, they said it appears that kids who watch lots of commercial TV may be developing a favorable "attitude toward consumerism and product acquisition."[34]

Children's demands often cause their parents to purchase the desired product. In two different studies, 85 to 90 percent of parents bought cereals, 50 to 60 percent bought snack foods, and 40 percent bought candies that their kids requested.[35]

Commercials on TV also prompt kids to ask to go to fast-food restaurants, according to a study by Atkin of fourth-through seventh-graders. Among heavy TV viewers, nearly half frequently asked to eat fast food. That compares to only one-fourth of kids who saw few TV commercials.[36]

So what if a child asks for a sugary cereal or to go to a fast-food restaurant? Parents have the right to say no, don't they? Indeed they do. But few want to tell their kids no time after time, day after day, month after month. Eventually, even the strongest-willed usually give in, rather than do battle with their children over and over again.

What Government Has—and Hasn't—Done

Over the years, two government agencies—the Federal Communications Commission (FCC) and the Federal Trade Commission (FTC)—have adopted rules to protect children from commercials or have considered doing so.

The FCC acted first. For example, in 1974 the FCC forced broadcasters to insert separators to help kids tell programs from commercials. It also effectively limited the amount of advertising during children's programs. It set the limits at 9.5 minutes per hour on weekends and 12 minutes per hour on weekdays.[37]

A decade later, the FCC got caught up in the deregulation frenzy that President Ronald Reagan brought with him to Washington. The commission, reoriented by the new Reagan appointees, decided to drop all limits on TV advertising, including the limit on advertising during children's programs.

To justify that 180-degree turn, the commission said that "marketplace forces can better determine appropriate commercial levels than our own rules." That rationale assumes the marketplace is a better regulator than the government and that if a station shows too many commercials, viewers will get disgusted and change the channel. Thus, economic forces will keep the number of commercials at reasonable levels.

The commission's theory has one major problem: There's no evidence to support it. No studies have shown whether adults will change the channel if a station shows too many commercials, University of California's Dale Kunkel said. And with young children, it's "conceptually flawed" to argue they'll switch channels "because we have very clear evidence that children below the age of about 5 lack the capability to discriminate programs from commercials," he said.

Action for Children's Television filed a lawsuit challenging the FCC's lifting of limits on advertising. In a sharply worded rebuke of the FCC, the U.S. Court of Appeals for the District of Columbia ordered the agency to review its decision.

The court said the FCC hadn't properly justified the new policy, particularly in light of its previous rulings. The court said that "[a]s the agency has seen it, kids are different; the Commission cannot now cavalierly revoke its special policy for youngsters without re-examining its earlier conclusions."[38]

The court didn't stop there. "For almost 15 years, the FCC's regulation of children's television was founded on the premise that the marketplace *does not* function adequately when children make up the audience," the court said. "The Commission has offered neither facts nor analysis to the effect that its earlier concerns over the market failure were overemphasized, misguided, out of date, or just downright incorrect. . . . Instead, without explanation, the Commission has suddenly embraced what had theretofore been an unthinkable bureaucratic conclusion that the market did in fact operate to restrain the commercial content of children's television" (emphasis in original).[39]

The court kicked the issue back to the FCC and told it to try again. The commission then sat on its hands. "The commission was clearly dragging its feet in response to the court's order," Kunkel said.

In 1988, Congress tried to take matters into its own hands by passing the Children's Television Act. The bill imposed limits on commercials, in addition to requiring broadcasters to provide educational and informational programming for children. Although Congress approved the bill, then-President Ronald Reagan pocket-vetoed it.

Congress was undeterred. It passed virtually the same bill in 1990. This time a new president, George Bush, begrudgingly allowed the bill to become law without his signature.

The bill, pushed by ACT and championed by Representative

Edward Markey (D-Mass.), should improve children's program-ming, though a 1992 study by the Center for Media Education found that some stations were claiming that cartoon shows, such as *The Jetsons,* constituted educational programming. Even the law's strongest supporters admit that it will change little about advertising. The bill's limits on commercials—10½ min-utes per hour on weekends and 12 minutes per hour on week-days—are the current norm among broadcasters. Kunkel said the limits "don't in any way reduce the amount of advertising that young children will be exposed to."

The FTC's Position

The Federal Trade Commission entered the fray in 1978, only four years after the FCC first imposed limits on kids' com-mercials. The FTC staff agreed with the FCC that children need special protection from advertisers. "It is both unfair and deceptive . . . to address televised advertising for *any* product to young children who are still too young to understand the selling purpose" of commercials or to evaluate them, the staff con-cluded (emphasis in original).[40]

The FTC staff also blasted those who advocate a free market with no restrictions on advertising to children. That position "assumes at least a rough balance of information, sophistication, and power between buyer and seller," the staff said. The staff said it's "ludicrous to suggest" that any such balance exists be-tween an advertiser who spends thousands per spot and a young child who may not understand a commercial's selling intent. Such a child "trustingly believes that the spot merely provides advice about one of the good things in life," the staff said.[41]

Even with children who are old enough to understand com-mercials, it's unfair to target them with ads that "induce them to take health risks" they can't evaluate, the FTC staff said.

Many food commercials do just that, the staff found and suggested that the FTC consider a set of strong remedies for solving the problems posed by children's commercials:

1. Ban all commercials either directed to or seen by "audiences composed of a significant proportion of children" under 8.
2. Ban commercials for sugared foods directed at children between 8 and 11 years old.
3. Require all advertisers of sugared food to fund nutrition and health information to balance their commercials.[42]

The FTC staff's proposal to ban all commercials aimed at kids younger than 8 was lauded and lambasted. Its far-reaching scope surprised everybody—both public-interest groups that supported some restrictions and industry groups that opposed any limits. Two public-interest groups—Action for Children's Television and the Center for Science in the Public Interest—had asked the FTC only to restrict commercials for candy and other high-sugar foods. They never dreamed the FTC staff would consider banning all commercials to young children.

Corporate America counterattacked with guns blazing. Peggy Charren, ACT's president, recalls that a "breathtaking coalition" of companies formed to fight the plan. "We had [every industry group] testifying that limiting advertising to children, that requiring disclosure and disclaimers, was going to do in these interests," she said. ACT claimed that broadcasters, advertising agencies, and manufacturers of children's foods and toys had amassed a $30 million war chest to fight the FTC.[43]

Industry's attack was multi-pronged. The opponents tried to stop the FTC from holding hearings, pressed Congress to bar the FTC from spending any money on the children's-television matter, and filed a suit challenging FTC Chairman Michael Pertschuk, among other actions.[44]

Nonetheless, the bureaucratic machinery cranked up and the FTC held six weeks of hearings. As the FTC moved closer to adopting a rule, though, Congress stepped in. The corporations couldn't get their way with the FTC, but they had enormous strength on Capitol Hill. Congress passed a law that it euphemistically called the FTC Improvement Act of 1980. The law stripped away the FTC's power to issue industrywide rules to stop *unfair* advertising practices, including advertising aimed at kids. It left the FTC with authority only to regulate ads on a case-by-case basis.

Elimination of its broad authority to stop unfair commercials destroyed the FTC's ability to restrict children's advertising. "Congress didn't want to tell the Federal Trade Commission they couldn't regulate advertising to children," Kunkel said. "I guess they thought it would be too unseemly. So they said, 'We think you're going too far with this new rule-making authority. We're therefore going to remove your authority to issue rules on unfair advertising.' That effectively unraveled the whole proceeding."

Just a few months later, Ronald Reagan was elected president. Virtually overnight, his appointees changed the FTC from an aggressive, consumer-oriented agency into a docile servant of business. One of the first issues on the new agenda was burying the children's advertising issue for good.

In 1981—the first year of the Reagan revolution—the FTC staff issued a new report. Once again, the staff said that commercials harm kids. But this time, instead of urging curbs on children's advertising, it recommended that the FTC drop the issue. The reason? The FTC could do nothing to solve the problems. The staff said "the record establishes that the only effective remedy would be a ban on all advertisements oriented toward young children, and such a ban, as a practical matter, cannot be implemented."[45] A ban was impractical, the staff said, because it would eliminate financial support for children's programs.

The staff's finding suited the new FTC commissioners just fine. In September 1981, they concluded that it was "not in the public interest" to continue the children's advertising rule making. "We seriously doubt . . . whether a total ban should ever be imposed on children's advertising . . . ," the commissioners said. "We cannot justify sacrificing other important enforcement priorities."[46] That effectively ended the FTC's role in regulating children's television advertising.

With governmental regulators safely out of the way, advertisers continued their use of unfair and deceptive practices. "The advertising practices to children are as bad as they've ever been," said Peggy Charren, who has monitored TV commercials for more than two decades. She blames that largely on the Reagan-led deregulation frenzy. Commercials to children really improved in the 1970s, Charren said, but the tide reversed in the 1980s. "Responsible children's advertising all but disappeared during Ronald Reagan's 'let 'em eat cable' administration," she told one interviewer.[47]

Solutions

Faced with government indifference toward television, advocates are taking various approaches to getting better food messages on children's TV.

In July 1991, the American Academy of Pediatrics, which represents 41,000 pediatricians, called for a ban on food commercials aimed at children, saying such commercials "promote foods that may have an adverse influence on children's health. . . . Obesity and elevated cholesterol levels are two of the most prevalent nutritional diseases among children in the United States, and television viewing has been associated with both."[48]

A month earlier, Secretary of Health and Human Services Louis Sullivan had endorsed changes in commercials targeting children. "I believe that a society that is concerned more about good health rather than a quick buck would not approve of industry advertising designed to increase our children's consumption of candy bars, sugary cereals, salty canned foods, and so on—products with minimal nutritional value," Sullivan said.[49]

Other advocates are working to persuade advertisers and TV stations to produce and run public service announcements (PSAs) promoting good nutrition. Representative Ron Wyden, chairman of the House Subcommittee on Regulation, Business Opportunities, and Energy, has been outspoken on this matter, as has the Center for Science in the Public Interest.

"Clearly, the industry needs to do a better job of self-policing," Wyden said. "I don't argue for elimination of these ads— or these products—just a little sensible balance." Wyden's goal: to have the "junk-food wasteland reseeded and nurtured with reasonable nutritional messages for our nation's youngsters."

In response to this new round of criticism, a few companies have responded. McDonald's developed a series of 12 PSAs on diet. CBS is donating 55 seconds each Saturday morning to run the spots. Dole, the fresh- and packaged-fruit giant, distributed a PSA that uses rap music to encourage kids to eat fresh fruits and vegetables. Other companies will likely develop PSAs, but the balance between PSAs and commercials is still tipped heavily in the direction of commercials.

The PSA idea isn't new. Way back in 1969, the White House Conference on Food, Nutrition, and Health recommended that food advertisers devote 15 percent of their advertising budgets to nutrition PSAs.[50]

Television stations often resist running more nutrition PSAs. They note that PSAs for a wide range of issues, including cancer, drug abuse, and AIDS all compete for a limited amount of air time. That's true. However, stations have a special responsibility to run nutrition messages because they make so much money marketing junk foods to kids. The least they can do is use the public airwaves to pass along some nutrition education to the public as well. And if there is enough pressure from angry parents, perhaps they will.

One rare exception to broadcasters' disinterest in nutrition is WLVI-TV, a major station in Boston. It and the Harvard Community Health Plan Foundation in 1992 ran "Janey Junkfood's Fresh Adventure," a 30-minute TV special developed by nutrition educator Barbara Storper, who also served as the irrepressible hostess. Rap music and snazzy graphics made this one of the neatest TV shows for kids ever made.

Another exception was a half-hour show produced by Consumers Union that ran on HBO in December 1992. The show, produced in a lively way guaranteed to keep kids' interest, exposed tricks used on labels and in ads to make foods appear much better than they are.

TV Programs

Many of the programs during which junk-food commercials appear offer another strong dose of poor nutrition to young viewers. The top-ranked comedies and dramas in 1988 contained nearly 10 references to food each hour, according to University of Minnesota researchers.[51] Usually, the foods that characters talked about or ate were non-nutritious.

Forty percent of the food references were to beverages such as coffee, alcohol, and soft drinks. Another 18 percent were to cookies, doughnuts, candy, ice cream and other sweets, and 7 percent were to salty snacks like chips and pretzels.[52] Thus, two-thirds of the foods eaten or mentioned were high in fat, sugar, or salt. Just under 10 percent of the food references were to fruits or vegetables.

Mary Story, one of the Minnesota researchers, noted that TV programs show "some of the worst aspects of the American diet." She and a colleague concluded that the "prime time diet is inconsistent with dietary guidelines for healthy Americans."[53]

What happens to TV characters who live on fatty, sugary foods? Absolutely nothing. That gives kids the message "that people are eating high-fat, high-sugar diets, but that there aren't any consequences," Story said. "People can eat whatever they want, but they're still thin."

Nearly all characters on prime-time television are slim, said Nancy Signorielli, associate professor of communication at the University of Delaware. "Even though there are so many references to unhealthy and fattening foods, as well as numerous instances of eating sweets, obesity . . . claims few victims on television," she wrote. This is particularly true of children and teenagers on TV, virtually none of whom are overweight.

The characters' slimness provides mixed messages about eating. "Television presents viewers with two sets of conflicting messages," Rutgers University professor Lois Kaufman wrote. "One suggests that we eat in ways almost guaranteed to make us fat; the other suggests that we strive to remain slim."[54]

All these messages particularly affect impressionable children, according to researchers from the Harvard School of Public Health and the New England Medical Center. They found that if a TV character eats potato chips, candy, or other non-nutritious foods, a child frequently does likewise while watching.

Television could easily improve its depiction of food and eating, according to Story and others. As evidence, they note that most television programs today don't glamorize smoking and drinking like they once did. "I think TV producers and the entertainment industry can play an important role in creating social norms and promoting healthy eating practices on television," Story said. "I think they have a social responsibility to promote the health of the nation."

CHAPTER 8

School Food

W hen he took away their Twinkies and Coke several years ago, Ken Maurer's students revolted. Maurer is superintendent of Metamora High School in Metamora Illinois, where lunch for most of the 800 students used to consist of cupcakes, chips, candy bars, and soft drinks. The junk foods were readily available—even the cafeteria sold them. Only about 120 kids ate the regular lunch daily. Most did so solely because they qualified for a free meal under federal guidelines.

Maurer became concerned that the high-fat, high-sugar lunches were harming the students' health, physical fitness, and behavior. "We noticed after lunch that kids were behaving in two ways," he said. "In some cases, they were hyper and seemed to have considerably more problems staying in seats and being quiet. On the other hand, we had kids who fell asleep, who didn't have the energy to make it."

Maurer tackled the cafeteria first. He didn't really blame the kids for shunning it. The cafeteria strove to cut costs by serving the cheapest food possible. The food was unattractive, portions were small, and there weren't any choices.

He started by eliminating junk food from the cafeteria's a la carte line. "Everybody told me, 'You're crazy—where you make your money is on the junk food,' " Maurer said. He also improved the regular lunches. The cafeteria started offering three entrees, at least two vegetables, a salad bar, soup, baked potatoes, and fresh fruit every day.

Despite these improvements, lots of kids still ate junk food for lunch because the student council store sold it. Maurer ordered the store to stop selling junk food during the school day. That's when the trouble began.

The student council, backed by the host of a radio talk show, started a boycott. Kids refused to eat in the cafeteria until the junk foods returned. The talk show host contacted Continental Baking Co., which sent a truckload of free Hostess Twinkies to the strikers. Another disk jockey, who backed Maurer, persuaded a local orchard to donate apples. News about the battle of wills reached as far away as England and Korea.

The boycott continued for most of a year. Maurer held fast, and the students' resolve eventually broke down. Today, about 600 kids—or 75 percent of the student body—eat in the cafeteria daily. "The kids think it's a great lunch," Maurer said. Perhaps most importantly, attendance and behavior have improved in the afternoon. In addition, the cafeteria—which used to lose up to $20,000 annually—now makes a small profit. Maurer gives the improved food all the credit.

Maurer is not alone in trying to improve school food. Across the country, many cafeteria managers are working hard to improve the nutritional quality of meals served to the 25 million students in the National School Lunch Program. Many schools, too, are enrolling in the federal School Breakfast Program, which helps 5 million kids get that all-important morning meal. And in June 1994, the U.S. Department of Agriculture

(USDA), which oversees the school food programs, proposed the first major improvement in decades. The proposal would set limits on the fat and saturated fat contents of meals.

Currently, though, most schools still ignore nutrition. Thousands of cafeterias serve hot dogs, hamburgers, french fries, nachos, ice cream, and other foods high in fat and sugar as part of the official school lunches. Many schools feature a la carte lines where choices are often limited to such items. Moreover, at more than 3,000 schools, the a la carte line also sells Taco Bell products, 800 schools offer Subway sandwiches, and 4,500 offer Pizza Hut pizza. Some schools have gone a step further, offering Pizza Hut pizza as part of the standard school lunch.

The food served in the cafeteria teaches children as much about nutrition as anything they learn at home or in class. "A lot of teachers feel like they can't stand up and talk about the essentials of a well-planned, heart-healthy diet when students go to the cafeteria and it's corn dogs and french fries," said Priscilla Naworski, director of the Healthy Kids Resource Center, which provides health-education materials to California teachers and cafeteria managers.

Increasingly, school cafeterias are becoming nutritional battlegrounds. The battle is clear in some cases, like when a school wants to let McDonald's take over the cafeteria. In others, though, the fight is more subtle. Frequently, it involves balancing what is ideal versus what is possible and practical.

In school cafeterias, the battles involve the nutritional quality of lunches, the offering of brand-name fast foods, the presence of non-nutritious foods that compete with cafeteria offerings, and school breakfast. We'll examine each of these issues in turn.

School Lunch

Most parents remember their school cafeterias with a shudder. Who could forget the mystery meat with pasty gravy, instant mashed potatoes, and canned vegetables that the cooks had seemingly boiled for days? And to top it off, the dried-out cake with Jell-O swirls?

Besides being unappealing, those lunches were clogged with fat, cholesterol, sodium, and sugar. Many of the meals got anywhere from 35 percent to 45 percent of their calories from fat. That's far above the 30 percent or less now recommended by health authorities.

Such meals aren't universal anymore. Today, the most successful lunch programs are the ones that offer the children choices. Progressive cafeterias, especially in large high schools, offer students up to ten entrees at every lunch, baked potatoes with toppings, salad and pasta bars, deli-style sandwiches, and lots of fresh fruit and vegetables.

Nevertheless, the U.S. Department of Agriculture's (USDA) own comprehensive study of school lunches, which was released in 1993, found that the nutritional quality of most was mediocre.[1] The researchers evaluated meals offered by 545 schools.

Meals averaged 38 percent of calories from fat. That's more than one-fourth more than is generally recommended. Only 1 percent of the schools offered meals that averaged under 30 percent of calories from fat. The lunches averaged 15 percent of calories from saturated fat, 50 percent higher than health authorities recommend. Only one out of the 545 schools offered lunches that met the guideline of 10 percent of calories from saturated fat.[2]

When it came to sodium, the schools did not do much better. The average lunch contained 1,479 milligrams. That's

The Downside of Free Food

UNDER THE NATIONAL School Lunch Act, schools get a certain amount of free food for each meal served. The USDA also gives schools "bonus" commodities it buys to support farm prices. Typically, 20 percent of the foods schools serve are USDA commodities.

Schools depend on those foods to help keep their lunch programs afloat financially. Unfortunately, many of the commodities are high in cholesterol, sodium, or sugar, and about half of all their calories come from fat, according to the Center for Science in the Public Interest.

Some of the foods provided in the largest quantities have included butter, Cheddar cheese, ground beef, lunch meat, ham, and eggs. Other foods include salted canned vegetables and canned fruit in heavy syrup.

Why does the USDA send schools commodities that are high in fat, cholesterol, sodium, and sugar? The answer dates back to 1946, when Congress created the National School Lunch Program, which it did primarily because half the men drafted in World War II had physical disabilities related either to childhood malnutrition or tooth loss.

But promoting good nutrition wasn't Congress' only goal. It also wanted to help farmers by providing more markets for excess foods they produced. Thus, the National School Lunch Program's purpose is to "safeguard the health and well-being of the Nation's children *and to encourage*

nearly two-thirds of the recommended maximum daily intake of 2,400 milligrams. (And remember, the National Academy of Sciences said that while 2,400 milligrams is recommended, 1,800 milligrams would be better.)

In 1990, the Center for Science in the Public Interest convened a Citizens' Commission on School Nutrition composed of nutrition and school food experts. The commission's White Paper encouraged the USDA to adopt nutrition standards for

the domestic consumption of nutritious agricultural commodities"
(emphasis added).

That dual purpose can cause
conflicts. When they occur, farmers usually win out over children.
As the non-profit Public Voice for
Food and Health Policy said in a
1989 report on fat in school
lunches: "The commodity distri-
bution program is basically designed to help the agricultural
community, and the products
which are purchased frequently
do not meet the nutritional needs
of school children."

Dairy products are the best
example. When overproduction
of milk pushes down prices, the
USDA steps in to help farmers by
buying milk until the price rises
again. Frequently, it processes the
milk into butter and Cheddar

cheese, two foods that are high in
fat, especially saturated fat. Then
it ships those foods to schools
across the country.

However, the USDA has
been improving the commodity
program by:

- Offering whole-wheat flour
  and brown rice.
- Reducing the amount of fat
  in ground beef and pork.
- Expanding the availability of
  fish, chicken, and turkey.
- Offering soybean oil to replace butter in cooking.
- Packing canned fruit in its
  own juice or light syrup instead of heavy syrup.
- Using less salt when processing vegetables.
- Barring processors from
  adding animal fats or tropical oils to commodity foods.

school lunches and to help school food service directors improve their meals. It urged that fresh fruits, fresh vegetables, and
legumes (beans, peas) be served much more frequently and that
relatively non-nutritious foods (soft drinks, candy, chips, and so
on) not be sold at schools at all. The White Paper also recommended that the fat content of lunches be limited first to 35
percent, then to 30 percent of calories, with no more than one-
third of the calories coming from saturated fat. It called for a

sodium limit of 1,000 milligrams immediately, then decreasing to 800 milligrams.[3]

In 1993 the USDA, reflecting the Clinton administration's concern about health, acknowledged problems with school lunches and vowed to fix them. Secretary of Agriculture Mike Espy wrote, "Eating habits based on sound nutrition are as essential as preventive medicine. Children's diets are too high in fat, sodium, and cholesterol and too low in fiber, fruits, and vegetables. We need to turn that around in the school lunchroom as well as at the family dinner table."[4]

Many cafeteria improvements, such as salad bars, offer students nutritious choices for lunch. Nutrition hasn't been the main impetus behind the changes, though. Instead, the meals have changed as food service directors struggled to persuade students to eat at school. With today's open campuses, many students—particularly those in high school—have the option of grabbing a burger at a nearby fast-food restaurant if they don't like the cafeteria food. To compete with these restaurants, many schools, besides offering the healthy options at lunch, have also opened a la carte lines that serve pizza, burgers, hot dogs, french fries, ice cream, and similar foods.

Most food service directors don't try to defend the nutritional quality of their a la carte foods. Instead, they argue that if the cafeteria doesn't serve fast foods, kids will simply go off campus for lunch.

Food service directors further contend—quite correctly—that they can't force kids to eat healthful foods. "About the best I can do is make it available and try to make it as good as I possibly can," said Dorothy Pannell, food service director for the Fairfax County Public Schools in Virginia. "But forcing our high school students, in particular, is not a viable alternative."

Pannell and her colleagues fear that offering only nutritious foods might cost cafeterias customers, something they can't afford, because nearly all of them must be self-supporting. "We have got to operate cost effectively," said Bob Honson, director of nutrition services for the Portland Public Schools in Oregon. "That's our number one goal. Our number two goal is to exemplify the U.S. dietary guidelines. It's a struggle sometimes to operate a program that's consistent with both of those goals. But I can guarantee that if we're not meeting the financial obligation of being self-sufficient, everything else that we do in terms of educating kids, serving nutritious foods, and all those things is going to go down the tubes."

Tami Cline, who was then the assistant director of food services for the Boston Public Schools, agreed. "We're under such tight financial constraints that unfortunately our number one concern becomes finances just to stay open," she said. "Then if we're operating in the black, we can start thinking about nutrition. That's the reality of it."

It's a theme echoed by food service directors nationwide, particularly in these tight economic times. Most food service directors—although not all—report that making lunches healthier raises costs. "Good nutrition doesn't always cost more, but sometimes it does," Cline said.

Elaine Keaton, food service director for the Albuquerque Public Schools, said a food supplier has developed a lower-fat hamburger patty she'd like to serve. But there's a catch: It costs eight cents more per patty than higher-fat versions. Eight cents doesn't sound like much—until you realize that Keaton serves lunch to 40,000 kids daily. The lower-fat version would cost Keaton an extra $3,200 each time she served it. That extra money doesn't exist in Keaton's budget, so she's forgoing the lower-fat patty. Instead, she's serving the regular hamburger patty with lower-fat foods to bring down the whole meal's fat level.

"These poor manufacturers are working their tails off with their research and development to come up with new products," said Keaton, "and then we're not ready to bite the bullet and pay for it."

Children Lose Out to Farmers

One of the most effective things schools could do to cut fat levels in lunches would not cost a dime. But federal law bars them from doing it.

The change? Stop serving whole milk.

A federal law requires schools to offer both low-fat milk and whole milk. Lots of food service directors want to stop serving whole milk, which gets half its calories from fat, to help cut fat levels in their lunches. Some also want to serve skim milk. But the USDA has decided that "low-fat" milk doesn't include skim milk.

Switching from whole milk to low-fat milk can significantly reduce a lunch's fat content. For example, a lunch of a hot dog, corn, a banana, and whole milk gets 33 percent of its calories from fat. If you switch the milk to 1 percent fat, though, the percentage of calories from fat drops to 27 percent. The saturated fat content drops from 15 percent to 11 percent.

The law is nothing more than a subsidy for dairy farmers. Dairies pay farmers based on their milk's fat level. The higher the fat, the more farmers make. But there also must be a market for that high-fat milk, which is where our children come in.

If schools stopped serving whole milk, the market for high-fat milk could decline. So Congress—pushed by the powerful dairy lobby—passed the law that turns schoolchildren's stomachs into a dumping ground for milk fat.

As this book was going to press, opposition to the milk law was growing in Congress. Senators Patrick Leahy (D–Vt.), Richard Lugar (R–Ind.), and Rep. Richard Durbin (D–Ill.) were leading efforts to repeal the measure.

The milk law is just one more example of what happens when farmers' financial interests compete with kids' nutritional interests: The farmers usually win.

Serving fresh fruits and vegetables also can raise costs. Frequently, schools can get free canned fruits and vegetables through the U.S. Department of Agriculture's commodity program. If they want fresh foods, though, they generally must buy them.

Some schools serve fresh fruits and vegetables despite the cost. Fairfax County has done so for years, and they're very popular with students. Depending on the season, Fairfax serves fruits such as apples, seedless grapes, oranges, bananas, melons, pears, and plums. One of the most popular vegetable offerings is veggie sticks with dip made from low-fat, low-sodium ranch dressing. The veggie stick assortment can include cauliflower, broccoli, carrots, cucumbers, and celery.

Cutting up all the vegetables increases preparation costs. "It's much easier to open a can or a frozen package," Pannell said. If Fairfax stopped serving fresh fruits and vegetables, Pannell said, it could cut lunch prices by about a dime.

In districts that don't already serve fresh fruits and vegetables, adding them can force food service directors to raise prices. They're loath to do so. That's because studies have found that each penny increase in the lunch price leads to a 1-percent drop in student participation.

To evaluate just how much it would cost schools to serve meals lower in fat and sodium, the USDA conducted a study in 1994. The results? Surprisingly, there was no difference in food costs between conventional meals and meals that met the goals for fat spelled out in the "Dietary Guidelines for Americans." (The study did not examine the costs of labor and equipment.)

Even considering the price of labor and equipment, many nutritional improvements in school lunches cost little or nothing. Here are some examples from schools around the country:

- Serve fresh fruits and vegetables as often as possible.
- Season cooked vegetables with herbs or lemon juice.

- Use frozen vegetables instead of canned ones whenever possible.
- Offer pasta bars, Mexican bars, taco salad bars, sandwich bars, picnic bars, and regular salad bars.
- Put leftovers from the main line on the bar.
- Use hamburger patties that are 15 percent or less fat by weight (some contain twice as much fat).
- Stretch ground beef by adding vegetable protein.
- Drain fat from ground beef after cooking, and then rinse the beef with water to remove yet more fat.
- Make spaghetti sauce with 50 percent ground turkey and 50 percent ground beef.
- Offer 1 percent fat milk and skim milk.
- Use 2 percent fat cottage cheese.
- Remove potato chips from the menu.
- Use soft margarine or vegetable oil instead of butter or shortening.
- Eliminate deep fryers; cook all foods by baking, roasting, or steaming to reduce fat.
- Reduce sugar in all recipes by 20 percent.
- Reduce salt in all recipes by 50 percent.
- Remove salt shakers from cafeteria tables.
- Use some whole-wheat flour, rolled oats, or other high-fiber flour in all baked goods.
- In most desserts, use egg whites instead of whole eggs.
- Serve baked desserts less often, and always offer fresh fruit as an alternative.
- Increase the use of unsweetened fruit juices.
- Discontinue the use of coconut.

Four small school districts in Minnesota incorporated those kinds of changes into LUNCHPOWER! meals in 1991. The fat levels of meals served at the 34 elementary schools that participated dropped from 40 percent of calories to 28 percent.

Balanced Meals Cost Less

Foods on a la carte lines usually cost students more than the traditional hot lunch, known as the Type A lunch. That's because the federal government only subsidizes Type A lunches.

The Type A lunch must be a complete, balanced meal that provides about one-third of the Recommended Daily Allowances for key nutrients. It must include specified portions of at least two vegetables or fruits; bread, pasta, rice, or other cereal grains; milk; and meat, poultry, fish, cheese, eggs, dry beans or peas, or peanut butter.

The U.S. Department of Agriculture bases its subsidy on whether the student gets a free lunch, pays a reduced price, or pays full price. Children qualify for free or reduced-price lunches based on their family income.

In the 1993–94 school year, the USDA gave school districts $1.725 for every lunch served to a student who qualified for a free meal. The USDA gave districts $1.325 for every reduced-price meal, and 16.5 cents for every full-price meal. In addition, schools receive free food, worth about 14 cents per meal.

Federal support for the National School Lunch Program has fallen way behind inflation, making it very difficult for schools to provide healthful, tasty meals. Current funding, adjusted for inflation, is only 58 percent of the initial 1946 funding level.

Source: Citizens Committee on School-Lunch Nutrition, *White Paper on School-Lunch Nutrition* (Washington: Center for Science in the Public Interest, 1990).

Student participation in the lunch programs didn't change at all. According to the University of Minnesota dietitians who conducted the study, an element crucial to the program's success was the enthusiastic support of the food service staff.[5]

Some states are helping school districts offer healthful

lunches. In Massachusetts, the state Education Department adopted a rule in 1988 requiring food suppliers to provide full nutrition information about their products. That includes levels of total fat, saturated fat, unsaturated fat, protein, carbohydrates, cholesterol, sodium, and calories.

The state publishes information supplied by the processors, and sends it to food service directors statewide. The state also helps directors interpret the numbers. "We work with them so they can use this information in making purchasing decisions," said Mary Jo Cutler, acting director of Massachusetts' Bureau of School Nutrition Services. "This makes it easier for the directors, and I believe they're purchasing more nutritious products as a result." Food service staffers praise the rule. Tami Cline in Boston said it is "instrumental" in helping districts offer more healthful lunches.

Clearly, it's possible for schools to produce a lunch that's at least somewhat lower in fat, cholesterol, sodium, and sugar. Moreover, many healthful changes don't raise costs. Yet a key question remains: Will kids eat the stuff?

The answer is a qualified "yes." Children can learn to love healthful lunches—if food service directors, cooks, teachers, and parents work together in educating them. The success of any changes hinges on how they're presented. The following seven factors are key:

1. Tackle the elementary schools first. The younger the children are, the more adaptable they'll be to changes in their food. By high school, many kids have been eating foods high in fat, cholesterol, sodium, and sugar for so long that it's tough to switch their diets.

2. Make the changes gradually. "You can't say, 'As of September 1 our meals are going to be 30 percent fat or less,'" said Keaton, the food service director in Albuquerque. "Kids won't accept it [if the food tastes different]. You have to evolve into it."

When Albuquerque decided to use whole-wheat flour in bread, the cooks started by using just 10 percent whole wheat. They gradually increased the level to more than 50 percent. When cooks make changes gradually, kids are less likely to object, or even notice what's going on.

3. As much as possible, adapt foods that kids already like instead of introducing new foods. Kids will probably accept a lower-fat hamburger patty—as long as it still tastes good. They may not even notice the change. But if cooks suddenly replace hamburgers with Chinese stir-fry over brown rice, the kids might revolt.

In Rochester, Minnesota, cooks found lower-fat versions of pizza and hot dogs that helped them cut fat levels in lunches below 30 percent. "The acceptance has been fine as long as we're modifying what they already like," said Sharon Hanson, the district's food service manager.

4. Involve kids in the changes. This may be the most important factor in changing meals. At Parson Hills Elementary School in Springdale, Arkansas, the PTA set up a "tasting table" in the cafeteria every two weeks. Students could taste healthful foods and then give their opinions about them. Foods that kids liked were added to the cafeteria menu.

Likewise, in Fairfax County, student panels conduct blind and non-blind taste tests of new products and recipes at least monthly. The product or recipe doesn't appear on the menu unless most students like it, Pannell said. A food approved by the panel rarely fails when cooks serve it to the whole student body. "I feel that the acceptability of our menus and our food has been greatly enhanced by the fact that students are involved," Pannell said.

5. Develop special promotions for healthy foods. High schools in Portland, Oregon, offer "training tables" targeted at student athletes, but available to all students. Foods served at the training table follow federal dietary guidelines. They're high in complex carbohydrates and low in fat. For example, the training table replaces the main line's french fries with baked potatoes.

Each school year, nutrition educators meet with every team to talk about how the training table can help athletes eat for optimal performance. The funny thing is that although nutritionists market the training table to athletes, many other students eat there, too. The reason: Student athletes have high status.

6. Integrate nutrition education in the curriculum with healthful changes in the cafeteria. Fran Shiffler, a parent activist, saw the importance of educating both teachers and students about good nutrition when cooks changed the meals at Parson Hills Elementary School. In addition to having the PTA offer food samples at tasting tables, some teachers discussed the changes and nutrition in the classroom. "In schools in the district where they just made the food improvements but did not have the nutrition education, there were complaints. I think nutritional awareness is key to acceptance," Shiffler said.

In Trumansburg Elementary School in upstate New York, some of the students were taught about bulgur, couscous, collard greens, and other relatively unusual and healthful foods. A few days after each lesson, which included geography, culture, and actual cooking, those foods were offered in the school cafeteria. David Levitsky, a Cornell University nutritionist, found that children who had learned about the foods ate between two and nine times as much of the foods as schoolmates who had not learned about them.

7. Encourage parents to offer healthful foods at home. "If you're going to change children's food habits, you need the assistance of the parents," said Peggy Burgess, the food service coordinator in Doddridge County, West Virginia. "Kids' food habits are pretty much in place by kindergarten."

Brand-Name Fast Foods in School Cafeterias

Increasingly, kids' food habits feature an almost slavish devotion to fast food. At the elementary level, most schools fight these habits by continuing to serve healthful lunches. As Pannell put it: "We very much play the role of mother."

By middle school and high school, though, thousands of districts have given up and are serving kids typical snacks and fast foods. They still serve traditional school lunches, but they also have a la carte lines that offer pizza, hot dogs, hamburgers, ice cream, nachos, potato chips, chocolate chip cookies, and similar foods of limited nutritional value. Not surprisingly, many food service directors are defensive about their a la carte lines.

Honson, the nutrition services director in Portland, admits that some kids always eat junk from the a la carte line. Honson said he fights this on a school-by-school basis.

A la carte lines aren't necessarily all bad. Many of them—including Honson's—offer nutritious choices in addition to their questionable offerings. Good lines offer salads, yogurt, bagels, fresh fruit, and healthy sandwiches.

Perhaps the most controversial item on a la carte lines is Pizza Hut pizza. By the start of the 1993–94 school year, Pizza Hut claimed it was serving about 4,500 schools nationwide.

The Suffield Public Schools in Connecticut greeted Pizza Hut with open arms. The district was serving frozen pizzas, but the kids didn't like them. That prompted Susan Fiore, director of food services, to call Pizza Hut. "In terms of nutrition, it falls right in line with our guidelines," Fiore said. "And in terms of student response, it was fantastic. The kids thought it was marvelous we had this name-brand product they recognized."

Compared to some other fast foods, Pizza Hut pizza is not

Chippers Get Crunched

Corporate efforts to inundate school cafeterias with foods of dubious nutritional value are nothing new.

In the late 1960s, potato chip manufacturers became defensive about nutritionists calling chips junk food. Adults responding to nutritionists' advice weren't eating as many chips. So the manufacturers decided to target children.

"As an industry, we are too often apologetic about the nutritional value of potato chips," said a top chip official at an industry meeting. "We need not be and should not be. On the contrary, we should extol the value of chips for their caloric content and energy value, *especially for youngsters*" (emphasis added).

What better way to reach kids than through school cafeterias? In 1972, the Potato Chip Institute International—an industry trade group—created an ad aimed at school food service directors. The ad, which ran in the *School Food Service Journal,* made the claim that a small bag of chips was more nutritious than an average-size apple.

The ad caused an uproar, since it was so blatantly deceptive. The Federal Trade Commission even entered the fray. It forced the PCII to sign a consent order agreeing not to use the apple-chip comparison again.

That didn't deter the chippers. The next year, they joined with the National Potato Foundation in a $200,000 ad campaign pushing the alleged nutritional value of potato chips. Again, a major goal was getting more chips into school cafeterias. An industry publication said schools "would provide an excellent avenue for increasing sales *and changing attitudes*" (emphasis added).

The industry's promotion efforts continue today. Despite them, however, more and more schools are dropping potato chips from menus because of their high fat content.

bad. Two slices from a medium pizza provide substantial amounts of calcium, protein, iron, and several B vitamins, in addition to modest amounts of vitamin C and fiber.

Yet Pizza Hut pizza is not a great food nutritionally. The crust is made with white flour, not fiber-rich whole wheat. Although Pizza Hut uses part-skim-milk mozzarella cheese, various types of the pizza get anywhere from 33 percent to 46 percent of their calories from fat, according to the company's information. Worse yet, two medium slices of Pizza Hut pizza contain 9 to 14 grams of saturated fat, which uses up 40 to 90 percent of a child's saturated-fat allowance for a whole day.

The pizzas also are extremely high in sodium. Two medium slices have from 867 milligrams to 1,648 milligrams of sodium, depending on the pizza type, which represents a hefty portion of a child's recommended daily allowance.

Fiore said she pushes plain and vegetable pizzas to help hold down fat levels. Pizza Hut pizzas are very popular with her students. At middle schools, between 60 percent and 70 percent choose Pizza Hut. At the high schools, 40 percent of the kids pick Pizza Hut for lunch. If the school board approves, Fiore wants to build a traditional school lunch—a meal with milk, fruit, and vegetable—around Pizza Hut pizza.

Initially, Fiore said, she was concerned that serving Pizza Hut would amount to brand-name advertising in schools. Then she realized the cafeterias already sold brand-name foods. "We have Columbo yogurt, Frito-Lay products, and so on," Fiore said. She added that kids associate quality with brand names. "If we switch from a Frito-Lay corn chip to Joe's local corn chip, the kids don't want to buy it because they recognize that Frito-Lay is a quality product and that's what they want," she said. "And it's the same sort of thing" with Pizza Hut.

The spirited defense of Pizza Hut by Fiore and some other food service directors is music to the ears of Roger Rydell, director of public affairs for Pizza Hut.

Rydell said Pizza Hut got involved in schools after food service directors approached the company looking for ways to keep their programs afloat. Rydell brushes aside concerns that schools serving Pizza Hut are assaulting students with brandname advertising, saying students "are extremely ·sophisticated and becoming more so," and that it's impossible to remove corporate references from schools. Baseball gloves, basketballs, pencils, textbooks, and other items students use in school carry brand names, he said.

"If you're going to eliminate any reference to corporate involvement in a child's education process, I would expect you'd have to lose a lot of branded names like Pyrex and Rand McNally," Rydell said. "It's one of those things that kids have become accustomed to. It isn't necessarily a nefarious sort of situation, especially when you put it in the context of all of the other products that they utilize in a given school day."

Arnold Fege, director of governmental relations for the National PTA, doesn't see it quite that way. He believes that letting Pizza Hut into cafeterias represents a relinquishment of public accountability and control in favor of the private sector.

"The question is: How far down are we going to want to compromise on nutrition?" Fege said. "I think that's the issue. I mean, who's next? Is McDonald's next? Is Burger King next? Is Domino's next? Are we going to set up competitions between the companies based upon the value of the product rather than the nutrition?"

A handful of schools—giving up on offering anything approaching a traditional, well-balanced lunch—have taken the next step that Fege fears. They've kicked out the school cooks and the National School Lunch Program, opting instead to let the local McDonald's franchisee take over the cafeteria.

One such school is the 1,300-student Fairview High School in Boulder, Colorado. Before the change, no more than 65 students and teachers ate in the cafeteria each day. Students didn't like the quality of the food or the service. "It was pretty evident we needed to make a change," said principal Don Groves.

The cooks resisted changes necessary to make their food more appealing, Groves said. The result: Lots of kids were leaving campus for lunch, and some weren't bothering to return for afternoon classes. "It really became an educational issue," he said.

So Groves got rid of the regular cooks and brought in the local McDonald's franchisee. (Two years later Boulder High School did the same.) The cafeteria began serving most of the McDonald's products, in addition to soup, salads, pizza, fresh fruit, and cereal. "This was not your basic McDonald's," said Tom Smith, dean of student activities. "There was a lot more than french fries and Big Macs."

Nonetheless, french fries and Big Macs are what the kids ate. "The staff ate the salad," Smith admitted. "The kids mostly ate the hamburgers."

By dropping out of the National School Lunch Program, Fairview lost federal reimbursement for free and reduced-price lunches served to low-income children. Fairview still offered subsidized lunches using the same guidelines as the federal government. But there's one slight catch: Kids qualifying for free meals had to take the foods chosen for them each day. Unlike other students, they got no choices.

The McDonald's franchisee provided the subsidy. Overall, the school broke even on the lunch program in the 1990–91 school year, while the franchisee lost some money.

Even with McDonald's moving in, only 350 kids ate the cafeteria lunch on an average day. That's about 27 percent of the students, far fewer than typically eat in a traditional, well-run high school cafeteria that offers choices.

Fairview's embrace of McDonald's didn't sit well with the Colorado Department of Education. "We'd like to see all the schools in the National School Lunch Program," said Dan McMillan, director of child nutrition for the department. Only schools in the program qualify for free commodities and federal reimbursements for free and reduced-price meals.

In addition, he said some Boulder doctors have complained about the nutritional quality of the McDonald's meals that Fairview and Boulder High School offer. "We were kind of hoping the pressure from the community itself would encourage the schools to go in the right direction," McMillan said.

By early 1994, the results of the McDonald's experiment were clear: The company decided to pull out of Boulder's high schools because it was still losing money, according to Nancy Paluk, the food service director for the area. The school system decided to run its own cafeteria.

Thornton High School in Thornton, Colorado, takes transforming the cafeteria into a fast-food court a step further. Students can choose among food from Chick Fillet, Taco Bell, and similar restaurants—without leaving the building. Other schools are doing the same thing.

Each day, students in the school's distributive-education program pick up pizza, burritos, candy bars, potato chips, and other items, said Mary Lou Burback, the director of nutrition services for the district. "There are no fresh fruits or vegetables. Nutrition is not a concern any more. They'll do anything for a buck." The students bring the food back to the cafeteria to sell. They also cook french fries and pump soft drinks. For this work, students get academic credit, but no pay.

Principal Max Willsey said he switched to fast food because students rejected "the potatoes and gravy syndrome" that dominated cafeteria meals. Only 60 students out of a total of 1,100 to 1,200 ate in the cafeteria before the change. Today, Willsey said, more than 300 students eat in the cafeteria each day. That's around 25 to 30 percent of the student body, again well below rates at schools with strong traditional lunch programs.

Willsey dismisses concerns about the lunches' nutritional quality. Healthful foods are available to students who want them, he said. For example, the cafeteria has a baked potato bar, salads, fruit, non-fat yogurt, and juice drinks. "As long as we have alternatives for them that are healthy, then I think it's their right to choose for themselves," Willsey said. But the kids simply don't eat the healthy alternatives, said Steve Urban, a teacher at Thornton. One reason for the lack of interest may be that the variety is so limited.

Willsey said the new lunch program, which debuted in the 1990–91 school year, meets all his goals. "Basically, you have a lot of free help, an atmosphere to stay on campus, and food that kids would normally eat anyway," he said.

After losing $15,000 to $20,000 annually with traditional lunches, Thornton's cafeteria now makes a profit of about the same amount, Willsey said. He predicted that other schools will follow Thornton's lead. "I have a variety of visitors here who can't wait to get into this kind of program," he said.

Let's hope he's mistaken about that. Schools that turn over their cafeteria to fast-food companies violate their duty to act *in loco parentis,* meaning "in the place of a parent." No responsible parent encourages his or her child to eat fast food for lunch every day. No responsible school should either.

But irresponsibility has even begun creeping into elementary schools. The fast-food bug has infected the three elementary and middle schools in Westchester, Illinois, a suburb of Chicago. The only lunches available to the 1,000 students come from McDonald's, KFC, and Domino's Pizza.

Turning the cafeteria over to McDonald's or replacing regular meals with a la carte lines can create serious problems for low-income children. At some schools that have stopped serving regular lunches, children who qualify for free or reduced-price meals may be able to choose from only a very limited variety of foods each day. Low-income students should have the same choices as everyone else. Schools also should be careful not to stigmatize low-income students by making them eat a special lunch each day. At Thornton High School, students who qualify for free or reduced-meal lunches can go next door to the middle school or have a bagged lunch delivered to the school.

The biggest fear is that schools that leave the National School Lunch Program will stop offering free and reduced-price lunches at all. By abandoning the federal lunch program, they lose their federal reimbursement for subsidized lunches and they are no longer obligated to provide subsidized meals. Unfortunately, for many poor kids the subsidized lunch at school is their only real meal of the day. To stop providing it would be unconscionable. Yet in these tough economic times, school districts are tempted to cut corners wherever possible.

Letting a fast-food chain take over the cafeteria sends three dangerous messages to students. First, it says there's nothing wrong with eating fast food every day of the week. The school, by offering fast food daily, endorses eating it daily. Second, the school implicitly gives its seal of approval to the food's nutritional quality. A school wouldn't serve food that was bad for students, now would it?

The third message is that the school will happily sell out its students to commercial influences if the price is right. Schools face tremendous financial pressures, but selling the students to the highest bidder is a crude way to balance the books. Schools—including their cafeterias—should be places of learning, not simply venues where fast-food giants can market to captive audiences.

Those companies are not simply trying to make a few more bucks around lunch time. They're seeking to hook kids on their brand names and products while they're young. Schools shouldn't help McDonald's or Pizza Hut do that.

Competitive Foods

It's bad enough that cafeterias have to battle with fast-food restaurants to attract students. Even worse, they frequently have to fight powerful forces within the school itself.

That's because principals, athletic departments, and student councils have discovered they can make lots of money selling soft drinks, chips, cupcakes, candy bars, and similar foods to students. "Everyone's in the food business, from the principal down to every club," said Keaton, the food service director in Albuquerque.

At most high schools—and some middle and elementary schools—banks of vending machines line the walls. In others, a student council–run store sells food. Usually, the machines and stores are stocked with junk foods. "The principals and the vending-machine companies don't always share our enthusiasm for nutrition," Honson, the nutrition services director in Portland, wryly observed. Honson and other food service directors hate vending machines because they compete with the cafeteria and undermine their pro-nutrition efforts.

Recognizing that, the Portland Board of Education passed a rule requiring schools to turn off vending machines during lunch. Another board policy says vending machines must offer students nutritious options. Honson said some schools still violate both rules. "At some schools, I'm convinced we're not going to make progress until the principal dies," he said.

Schools that allow vending machines or student stores to sell junk foods do more than promote bad eating habits. As the South Carolina School Food Service Association put it: "The sale of these foods of minimal nutritional value sends a message to students that it is acceptable to compromise health for monetary gain."

In 1980, the U.S. Department of Agriculture sought to limit

sales of junk foods at schools. It adopted a regulation that barred schools from selling soft drinks, gum, and hard candy before the last lunch period ended.

In 1984, though, the National Soft Drink Association filed a suit challenging the regulation. A federal appeals court sided with the industry. It ruled that the USDA lacked the legal authority to ban competitive foods throughout schools and at times other than lunch. The court said the USDA could just bar competitive foods from the cafeteria—and only during lunch. The ruling paved the way for vending machines to invade schools once again and challenged local school systems to control the sale of competitive foods.

Some local districts and states have adopted their own restrictions on foods that compete with cafeteria meals. The state of Maryland, for instance, bars the sale of soft drinks, gum, and other sugary junk foods outside or inside the cafeteria from the beginning of the school day to the end of the last lunch period.

Mary Klatko, director of food and nutrition service for the district, also controls all the vending machines in the schools. She stocks them with fruit juice.

The Kentucky Board of Education adopted a policy like Maryland's, but over strong protests by principals who relied on vending-machine sales to support extracurricular activities. The rule bans the sale of competitive foods until 30 minutes after lunch ends.

"You had a number of school administrators who were scheduling breaks in the morning for the express purpose of running the kids by the machines," said Paul McElwain, director of school food services for the Kentucky Department of Education. McElwain said the number of students eating lunch at school rose 2 percent in 1990–91, when the ban took effect. "You've got 11,000 more kids eating [a school] lunch every day," McElwain said. "That's 11,000 kids that are better prepared to learn something in the afternoon."

West Virginia has one of the oldest competitive food rules. The policy, which took effect in the 1976–77 school year, bars schools from selling soft drinks, candy, gum, and flavored ice bars any time during the school day.

Principals and vending companies have twice tried to get the rule overturned, said Harriet Deel, director of child nutrition programs for the state Department of Education. The state board of education rejected the pleas both times.

However, many schools still have vending machines, stocking them with foods ranging from juice, fruit, popcorn, and peanuts to beef jerky, potato chips, and cookies. West Virginia's rule is seriously flawed, but it is a step in the right direction.

Deel said principals and student clubs have found they can make "substantial revenues" selling healthful foods. The only drawback: Profit margins are lower than for junk foods.

In states where there are no laws governing vending machines, getting rid of them can be difficult. In addition to student and principal pressure, there can be commercial pressure, especially in the case of soft-drink vending machines. That's because the cola companies have bought their way into the schools by donating scoreboards and other equipment. Many schools feel obligated by the gifts. "When they've accepted lots of things from these companies, it's hard to turn around and take the machines out," said Vivian Pilant, director of food services for the South Carolina Department of Education.

In Fairfax County, Pannell welcomes vending machines instead of fighting them. A vending machine is "no worse than the food you put in it," she said. She stocks them with healthy foods like salads, bagels with cream cheese, cereal with milk, and popcorn. She hasn't totally won the war, though, because some machines still contain junk foods. "I tried to eliminate potato chips, and I got petitions on napkins," Pannell said.

The Importance of Breakfast

For generations, parents across America have nagged their kids to eat breakfast. "Breakfast is the most important meal of the day," they've proclaimed.

Millions of kids, too sleepy and rushed to bother with food in the morning, have ignored their parents' claims. According to the American School Health Association, half of the girls and one-third of the boys in the eighth and tenth grades had not eaten breakfast on five or more days during a typical week.[6] The Bogalusa Heart Study found that one out of six 10-year-olds skipped breakfast, and that many of those who ate at home had dined on cake, colas, or other junk food.

The most compelling evidence that breakfast is important comes from a 1989 study of poor third- to sixth-graders in Lawrence, Massachusetts. Researchers tracked the children twice: before and after their schools signed up for the national School Breakfast Program. Under the breakfast program—just like the lunch program—the USDA subsidizes school meals.

The results were clear: Students who ate breakfast at school performed better than students who did not. Although, the gap wasn't enormous, in some cases it meant the difference between success and failure. In addition, kids who ate breakfast at school had less tardiness and better attendance than kids who did not.[7]

Dr. Alan Meyers, the director of the study and assistant professor of pediatrics at the Boston University School of Medicine, admits his study isn't perfect scientifically. That's because the researchers couldn't control variables besides breakfast that might have affected students' school performance. Nonetheless, he believes it and other studies provide persuasive evidence that eating breakfast affects whether a child succeeds in school. He also believes schools shouldn't require iron-clad scientific proof of a

breakfast program's benefits before starting one. "We have sufficient evidence to suggest it's the right thing to do from a policy
perspective and an education perspective," he said.

The staff of a congressional subcommittee agreed with Dr.
Meyers. It said the "limited research" conducted on the relationship between hunger and learning "points to several non-
controversial conclusions." These include:

- Children who eat a morning meal are better able to handle complex tasks, make fewer errors, are more attentive,
  participate more, and are more likely to ask questions.
- Children who don't eat breakfast get sluggish in the late
  morning.
- Hungry children don't learn as efficiently as well-fed children.[8]

Principals and food service directors around the country
have no doubts that eating breakfast greatly affects students' behavior and performance. Shirley Watkins, then director of nutrition services for the Memphis Public Schools, started a
limited breakfast program in the 1960s. "We saw some real
changes in the children who participated in the breakfast program," she said. "They were able to achieve in the classroom,
they were not as lethargic, they were more responsive to the
teacher, and attendance improved." Today, Memphis offers
breakfast in all but two of its schools.

Memphis started its breakfast program before the federal
government stepped in to help school districts. It wasn't until
1966—20 years after the National School Lunch Program
started—that Congress approved the School Breakfast Program
as a pilot project. The aim was to provide breakfast to poor children and those who had long bus rides to school.

The program was such a success that Congress expanded it
nationwide and made it permanent in 1975. Under the law, any

school district can obtain a federal subsidy for its breakfast program. As with the lunch program, the subsidy is larger for breakfasts provided to low-income students for free or at a reduced price. In the 1993–94 school year, the federal government gave districts 96 cents for each free breakfast, 66 cents for a reduced-price breakfast, and 19 cents for a full-price meal. School districts with a large number of low-income children get an additional 18.25 cents per meal. Some school districts find that the federal reimbursement allows them to make a small profit on breakfast. They then use this money to subsidize their lunch programs.

To qualify for federal reimbursement, the breakfast must include bread, cereal, or meat; a fruit, vegetable, or juice; and milk. The USDA also urges schools to offer protein-rich foods such as eggs, meat, fish, cheese, and peanut butter as often as possible.

The guidelines give schools great flexibility. They can offer as simple or as elaborate a breakfast as they like. Even schools without cooking facilities can set out cereal, milk, and juice and still get the federal subsidy.

With all the evidence supporting breakfast, it seems as if every school in the nation would serve it. Unfortunately, more than half do not. Partly because so few schools offer breakfast, just over 5 million students eat breakfast at school. That contrasts with the more than 25 million who eat lunch.

Schools that don't offer breakfast short-change all their students, but particularly those from low-income families. For many poor students, a school breakfast program means the difference between eating or not eating in the morning. Overwhelmingly, students who take advantage of school breakfasts are poor. In 1990, nearly 86 percent of students eating breakfast had family incomes low enough that they qualified for free or reduced-price meals. By contrast, just 46 percent of students eating lunch received free or reduced-price meals.

Offering breakfast is a basic fairness issue, said Ed Cooney, deputy director of the Food Research and Action Center (FRAC) in Washington, D.C. FRAC has worked with schools around the nation to start breakfast programs.

"There's not equal educational opportunity if a kid has breakfast at home or gets breakfast at school, and you're a poor kid who goes to a school that doesn't offer breakfast," Cooney said. The breakfast program could become one of the key educational issues of the decade, Cooney predicted.

Support for the School Breakfast Program is far from universal. Opponents' primary contention is that breakfast should be a family meal served at home. However, the reality is that poor families sometimes lack the money to serve breakfast. Even in better-off families, morning schedules can make it impossible for families to eat together.

Closely related is a philosophical objection that serving breakfast isn't an appropriate role for schools. Cooney dismisses that concern. "If you accept the principle that there's a relationship between nutrition and learning—and you'd have to be brain dead if you didn't—then it is a proper role for a school," he said. "If you want to have higher test scores, you ought to be a major proponent of the School Breakfast Program."

Some school officials claim that it's too much trouble to offer breakfast, contending they'd have to rearrange bus schedules, hire more cooks, and solve myriad other problems. Many of those problems are real. However, school districts around the country are showing they all can be overcome and that doing so is worth the trouble, though not every district pays much attention to nutrition. Here are a few examples:

• In rural Doddridge County, West Virginia, 98 percent of the students ride buses. That makes having a breakfast program critical—and very popular. Every morning the Doddridge schools offer kids at least three cold cereals, some type of bread, at least three juices, milk, various hot dishes, and fresh fruit, usually including apples, grapes, bananas, and oranges. They try to offer strawberries, nectarines, peaches, cantaloupe, and kiwi when they're available and affordable. For many students, it's their first exposure to kiwi, a fruit rich in vitamin C.

Before the breakfast program started, principals scheduled study halls or library periods during the last half hour before lunch. The reason? Kids were too hungry to concentrate. Now, lessons can continue right up to lunch. That made believers out of principals, according to Peggy Burgess, the district's food service coordinator.

• In Springdale, Arkansas, food service director Marilyn Huffman helps hold down labor costs by putting foods on a "breakfast bar" where students serve themselves. Besides saving money, the bars are popular. "I think they enjoy being able to select their own foods," Huffman said. All schools—elementary, middle, and high school—have breakfast bars.

The food choices differ from school to school. Besides cold cereals, the bars can have eggs, muffins, French toast, sausages, whole-wheat bread, pancakes, breakfast casseroles with meat, and hash browns.

• At North Hardin High School in Kentucky, the cafeteria is off the beaten path. Only about 60 of the school's 1,100 students trekked to it for breakfast each day. So Jamey Kizer, food service director for the Hardin County Public Schools, decided to try taking the food to the students.

Kizer bought two carts. Each morning, cooks load them with cinnamon rolls, muffins, fruit, sausage-and-egg biscuits, juice, milk, and other foods that kids can eat with their hands. Then they roll the carts to the school's two main entrances and sell food to kids walking through the doors.

Today, between 200 and 300 kids eat breakfast every day. "We have found that when the food is there, they eat," Kizer said. The number of kids eating the regular cafeteria breakfast also rose. Kizer thinks that may be because the carts remind kids of food when they walk into school.

A growing number of states, impatient at the slow growth of breakfast programs, are passing laws requiring at least some schools to offer them. Commonly, the laws require schools to offer breakfast if a certain percentage of students is poor enough to qualify for free or reduced-price lunches. About a dozen states now have such laws.

West Virginia's law is one of the broadest in the nation. Passed in 1981, it requires all public schools to offer breakfast unless they get a waiver from the state. Waivers are rare; only five schools have received them.

To back up the breakfast law, the state board of education requires that students get at least ten minutes to eat after arriving at school. Any district that violates the rule—which the state enforces fiercely—can lose its accreditation.

The law works. Because of it, for example, almost one in four students got breakfast each day in October, 1993. In one Wyoming county almost half the students were getting breakfast. School officials there say mornings now go more smoothly, and that the breakfast program has reduced skipping, tardiness, and irritability.

The USDA, after years of inaction, also is starting to push schools to offer breakfast. Such active promotion was "an unheard-of event in the eighties," said Cooney, the deputy director of FRAC. In 1990, the USDA announced it would give school districts $23 million in grants over five years to help them start breakfast programs. Backers of the breakfast program said the grants will give a big push to expanding it. In 1994 Senator Patrick Leahy (D-Vt.) was pressing for additional financial assistance to schools.

Nonetheless, tens of thousands of schools still don't serve

breakfast. That handicaps their students who either can't or won't eat breakfast at home. Every school that serves lunch also should serve breakfast—no ifs, ands, or buts.

Expanding the breakfast program is a difficult, district-by-district process. Parents can play a big role. Around the country, parents—working either with the local PTA or a national group like the Food Research and Action Center—have convinced school officials to start breakfast programs. In Chapter 11, we'll explain how you can work to get a breakfast program in your child's school if it doesn't offer one.

Cause for Optimism

As this book was going to press in mid-1994, change was in the air. Senator Leahy had introduced legislation that would limit the fat content of school meals, repeal the requirement that schools offer children whole milk, encourage states to limit junk foods, and even provide small amounts of organic foods to schools. At the same time, the USDA, using its existing authority had been pressing for some of those same goals. Perhaps soon school meals will be considerably more healthful.

CHAPTER 9

Corporations Invade the Classroom

The sixth-grade class is in the midst of a unit on nutrition and fitness called "Balancing Your Act." To test the students' knowledge, the teacher hands out an activity sheet. He instructs the kids to match nutrition and fitness terms with their definitions.

A student trying to match the word "fats" with the given definitions could have a hard time. That's because the correct definition, according to the teacher's guide, is "nutrients that supply energy and help insulate the body." The "definition" makes fat sound like a swell substance kids should eat in large quantities.

Unfortunately, the definition doesn't mention that some fats clog arteries and cause other health problems—some of which start in childhood. Nor does it mention that all major health authorities recommend that sixth-graders and everyone else over age 2 limit fat in their diets.

Next, the teacher hands out reprints from *Sports Illustrated for Kids* that are part of the "Balancing Your Act" program. These include two full-page McDonald's ads. One quotes Jackie

Joyner-Kersee, the Olympic runner, as saying: "The only time I stop is when I'm biting into a Quarter Pounder."

The ad copy continues: "Not even Jackie Joyner-Kersee can move fast without the right fuel. And great fuel for fast movin' includes food high in protein and carbohydrates. Like a Quarter Pounder with Cheese sandwich. Grab one for lunch and you'll also get lots of calcium, iron, and vitamin A—all important nutrients for a healthy body. But don't go overboard on any one kind of food, not even a Quarter Pounder. 'Cause to keep your body running smooth, you need a variety of other healthy food and lots of exercise."

Nowhere does the ad mention that a Quarter Pounder with Cheese gets 49 percent of its calories from fat. Small print does admit the sandwich has a whopping 28 grams of fat, but doesn't put this number in any context. For a typical child who eats 1,800 to 3,000 calories daily, the sandwich supplies between one-third and one-half of his or her daily fat and saturated fat quota. The sandwich also has about half of the sodium (1,090 milligrams) and more than one-third of the cholesterol (115 milligrams) that a child should eat in an entire day. The ad indicates that a Quarter Pounder is a healthful food. It clearly is not.

Trading cards included with the reprints feature sports stars. Each card has a "nutrition tip" on the back. Here's one: "McDonald's menu has a variety of wholesome, basic foods like meat, bread, dairy products, and vegetables. Now that's balance!" That's a nutrition tip?

Who created these so-called nutrition education materials? Not surprisingly, it's McDonald's. What is surprising is that the company has the nerve to charge $17.90 for the unit.

What's going on here? How can blatant misinformation and corporate propaganda end up in classrooms? The answer lies in three related problems: the poor quality of nutrition education in schools, the funding crisis in many school systems, and the corporate invasion of America's classrooms.

Unfortunately, lots of schools still offer little or no nutrition education. Some teachers consider nutrition education a luxury, something that competes for class time with reading, writing, and arithmetic. In addition, many teacher training programs lack nutrition units. It's hardly fair to expect teachers to tackle a subject they know little about.

To fill the void, some teachers rely on "nutrition education" materials offered by food companies like McDonald's or producer groups like the National Dairy Council. Not surprisingly, those materials promote the sponsor's view of nutrition—and consumption of the sponsor's products.

How the Government Dropped the Ball

A decade ago, the General Accounting Office (GAO), the investigative arm of Congress, found that nutrition education was a hit-or-miss affair in the nation's schools. "Although the support has increased and the status of nutrition education has improved . . . nutrition education remains basically unstructured, sporadic, and a low priority," the GAO said in 1982. ". . . [State] officials responsible for nutrition education told us that teachers' knowledge of and interest in nutrition largely determine its importance in the classroom."[1] Unfortunately, that finding is just as true today as it was then.

There are so many people to blame for this sorry state of affairs that it's hard to know where to start. But the federal government is a prime culprit.

In 1977, Congress created the Nutrition Education and Training Program (NET) to improve nutrition education for students, teachers, and cafeteria workers. Congress appropriated

50 cents for every student in the nation, or about $25 million annually. The USDA gave the money to the states, which used it to develop classroom lessons, conduct in-service sessions for teachers, and train cooks.

Then Ronald Reagan took office. At his behest, Congress slashed the budgets of all child nutrition programs, including NET. It cut NET's funding to $5 million annually, forcing states to dramatically reduce their nutrition education efforts. In 1994, Congress finally pushed NET's funding to $12.4 million. That's still less than half of the original funding, though the Clinton administration requested an additional $18.4 million to wage a media campaign aimed at children in 1995.

States, facing their own financial problems, haven't closed the funding gap left by the NET cuts. Only nine states provide funds for nutrition education, according to a national survey conducted by researchers at Pennsylvania State University.[2]

Many states don't require prospective teachers to have any training in nutrition. Out of 41 states that responded to the Penn State survey, only 20 require future health teachers to take a nutrition course. On the other hand, 39 of the 41 states require future home economics teachers to take a nutrition class.

An even more telling indication of nutrition's low priority in the educational system is the fact that only 30 states require schools to teach it at some grade level. The remaining states only encourage schools to include nutrition in the curriculum.[3]

The Corporate Curricula

While the government has failed to adequately promote nutrition in the schools, corporations have invaded American classrooms like never before. Food companies are some of the most aggressive interlopers.

In recent years, at least 75 food-related corporations or in-
dustry associations have offered materials to schools. They in-
clude the Almond Board of California, Chef Boyardee, Gerber,
Hershey Foods, the National Hot Dog & Sausage Council,
Pillsbury Co., the Salt Institute, the Sugar Association, and the
Washington State Apple Commission, among others.

Food manufacturers and producer groups flood teachers
with free or inexpensive pamphlets, games, film strips, movies,
and other materials. Some provide entire nutrition curricula for
preschool through high school. Others send product samples to
home economics teachers, give schools money based on the
number of food labels students collect, or give scoreboards to
schools that accept their vending machines. And some advertise
directly to students on *Channel One,* a television program that's
broadcast to thousands of classrooms.

Food companies' favorite ploy is to send teachers "educational" materials for classroom use. There would be nothing
wrong with this if the materials were purely educational, but
most are little more than ads cloaked in the robes of educational
respectability. A House subcommittee chairman, Representative
Frederick Richmond, summed up the situation in 1977: "Aware
that government has not taken an active role in providing nutrition education in our school systems, food companies and trade
organizations are filling the void. Under the guise of nutrition
education, they are promoting their products to captive audiences of children."[4] Alas, his message still rings true today.

Tight budgets make schools especially vulnerable to corporate assaults. "Schools' chronic funding shortages lead teachers
to welcome free education materials," said a report by Consumers Union, the publisher of *Consumer Reports* magazine.
"Unable to win sufficient public funding for their educational
role, schools are turning into an advertising medium."[5]

Twenty million students use corporate-sponsored teaching
materials annually, according to Consumers Union. Two mil-

lion students receive product samples and coupons in school. And "countless millions more" see TV commercials and magazine ads in the classroom.

What motivates corporations to help schools? It is possible that some companies feel twinges of social responsibility. Their overriding concern, though, is hooking customers. What better place to do it than a school, where there's a captive audience and teachers can reinforce and legitimize the message? Studies in both the United States and Scandinavia show that "schools and teachers lend authority and approval to the sponsoring company and to the company's message," said a study by the International Organization of Consumers Unions.[6]

Companies' real motive for providing educational materials comes through loud and clear in an ad by Lifetime Learning System, which develops classroom materials for corporations.

"School is . . . the ideal time to influence attitudes, build long-term loyalties, introduce new products, test market, promote sampling and trial usage, and—above all—to generate immediate sales," the ad said.[7] Another ad in *Advertising Age* tempted companies with this message: "Kids are big spenders. . . . Kids spend 40% of each day in the classroom where traditional advertising can't reach them. Now you can enter the classroom through custom made learning materials created with your specific marketing objectives in mind."

So just how bad are corporate-sponsored materials? Consider "Around the World with Beatrice/Hunt-Wesson Inc.," a home economics program that ostensibly teaches students about ethnic foods and nutrition.

The "program objectives" listed in the teacher's guide make the company's motives clear. The first goal is "to introduce students to Beatrice/Hunt-Wesson Inc. products." Five out of six activity masters for students have pictures of the company's products and prominently feature brand names. In addition, between one and four Beatrice/Hunt-Wesson products are listed as ingredients in each of the 32 recipes included.

One lesson, called "Welcome to Rosarita," allegedly teaches students about the foods of Puerto Rico, Cuba, and Mexico. It just happens that "Rosarita" is the name of a Beatrice/Hunt-Wesson line of Hispanic foods. The activity master for students says: "Some Hispanic foods available throughout the United States today include the Rosarita line of products. . . ."

Another lesson, called "Oil: Now You're Cooking" pushes students to use lots of vegetable oil. Of course, Beatrice/Hunt-Wesson produces a major line of oils. As part of the lesson, teachers are urged to have students "discover the cuisine of their own ethnic backgrounds" by finding four recipes that origi-nated in the country of their heritage. There's only one surpris-ing coincidence: Every recipe includes oil.

While extolling the virtues of cooking oil, the lesson never mentions that oil is 100 percent fat. There's nary a word about obesity and other dangers of high-fat diets.

We called Hunt-Wesson to ask why this information isn't in-cluded. "This is not a nutritional program," said Kay Carpen-ter, Hunt-Wesson's manager of corporate communications. "It's a program to teach children how to shop for and to plan for and to prepare meals. There's a definite place for nutritional educa-tion, but these were not developed for that purpose."

Oh? The teacher's guide instructs teachers to tell their stu-dents that "as part of a balanced diet, fats provide a concen-trated source of energy (more than twice as much in a gram of fat as in a gram of carbohydrate)." It also instructs them to say that fats and oils provide essential fatty acids and that fats help the body use fat-soluble vitamins. Isn't that nutrition education?

There was a long pause while Carpenter read the teacher's guide. "I see where that does provide some nutritional informa-tion," she added. Then she tried another tack: "We don't have anything like this that we send out any longer," she said. "These are outdated materials."

Oh? A teacher we know got them from Hunt-Wesson only a couple of months before the interview.

Carpenter shifted gears again. This unit is still available if teachers specifically request it, she said.

Oh? The teacher we got it from simply wrote to Hunt-Wesson asking for nutrition education materials. The teacher didn't request the specific unit.

"I don't know the specific instance" is all Carpenter could say. Then she circled back to try again. The program dates from 1986, Carpenter said, and doesn't mention fat's drawbacks because fat wasn't a major dietary issue then. "The issue with the fat and the fat labeling is something that really has come up within the last year," she said.

That's not true, either. In 1977, the Senate Select Committee on Nutrition and Human Needs urged Americans to cut their fat intake to less than 30 percent of total calories. In 1979, the U.S. Surgeon General also recommended that Americans limit fat in the diet. And in 1980, a pamphlet entitled "Dietary Guidelines for Americans"—jointly issued by two federal departments—said Americans should avoid too much fat.

Carpenter defended the program as "a very legitimate teaching aid" despite its listing of Hunt-Wesson products in every recipe. "They don't need to use our products necessarily to come up with a good recipe," Carpenter said. "We're not trying to do anything subversive in the classroom, that's for sure."

Carpenter's comments are a classic example of the fancy footwork many corporations engage in when asked about their "education" programs.

A popular tactic is to claim, as Carpenter did, that the company isn't distributing a particular program anymore. A Kraft spokeswoman took this tack when we called to ask about the "American Taste, Cheese in the Melting Pot" program it sells to teachers for $12.

It's little wonder the spokeswoman didn't want to discuss the program. Pictures of Kraft products and references to them dominate the film strips, recipes, and student activity masters.

Basically, the unit is one long promotion of process cheese. It includes a film strip titled "The Process Cheese Story." The film strip script begins: "Ever wonder who invented those process cheese slices that you love in your sandwiches?" The answer, of course, is Kraft's founder. The script concludes that process cheese is "economical, wholesome, and versatile. For many reasons, it's an American favorite." Kraft even includes a packet of emulsifier so students can make process cheese in class.

The film strips and student materials don't say a word about the high fat and sodium levels in most cheeses. However, the teacher's guide devotes more than a page to the protein, minerals, calcium, and other nutrients in cheese. The guide admits "some fat-modified cheese products are now available," but said that dietary fat is necessary "for providing energy and transporting fat-soluble vitamins..."

That is propaganda, not education. Charging teachers $12 for it is the height of chutzpah.

As the Hunt-Wesson and Kraft examples show, what companies leave out of their "educational" materials is often more important than what they put in. That is nowhere more true than in some of the school materials created by the National Dairy Council.

The NDC has been prodding schoolchildren to drink milk and eat other dairy products for more than 70 years. It has been active in schools longer than any other producer group or food company. "It used to be they were the only show in town," said Isobel Contento, who coordinates the nutrition education program at Columbia University's Teachers College.

The NDC has offices in cities around the country that distribute materials and conduct influential teacher-training workshops. For example, a Minnesota study found that from 1977 to 1985, 85 percent of the state's school districts used NDC curriculum materials. Seventy-five percent of the state's pre-schools did likewise.[8]

Many teachers like the NDC because it provides complete nutrition curricula for preschoolers through senior high school students. All the materials are bright, lively, and professionally produced. But for years, they've largely ignored the connection between fatty diets and serious health problems.

They've also ignored advances in nutrition education. The NDC materials clung tenaciously to the Basic Four even after it was obsolete. You remember the Basic Four—you probably learned it in elementary school. Its concept is simple: To be healthy all you need to do each day is eat a certain number of dairy products; fruits and vegetables; grains and cereals; and meat or so-called meat alternates like fish, chicken, eggs, peanut butter, and beans. Government health officials, along with the dairy and meat industries, developed the Basic Four in the 1940s and 1950s as part of the fight against malnutrition. Back then, the concern was that Americans weren't eating enough food. Today, the concern is very different. Too many Americans are eating too much, particularly of foods high in fat, cholesterol, sodium, and sugar. Nevertheless, the Dairy Council still pushes the Basic Four since it emphasizes the need to eat plenty of dairy products.

It's not as if there haven't been alternative nutritional guidelines available for years. "Dietary Guidelines for Americans," issued by the USDA and the Department of Health and Human Services, has been around since 1980 and provides detailed information on choosing food for everyone age 2 and above. It stresses the need to choose a diet lower in fat and saturated fat—two substances found in large amounts in most dairy products.

And in April 1992, the U.S. Department of Agriculture replaced the Basic Four with the Food Guide Pyramid. The pyramid shows graphically what foods people should eat and in what proportions. The meat and dairy industries were extremely upset by the new guidelines because the pyramid advises that their foods make up only a small proportion of the diet, emphasizing that breads, cereals, rice, pasta, fruits, and vegetables should be the dominant components.

So it's not hard to understand why the dairy council has continued to cling to the Basic Four for as long as possible. "Eating a variety of foods from the Four Food Groups can help you get all the nutrients you need," says the student booklet for the secondary school curriculum.[9]

The booklet, which was being phased out in 1994, has only a brief section on fat. Some foods, "such as spareribs or avocado," are naturally high in fat, according to the booklet. It doesn't mention that most dairy products also are naturally high in fat. It's a rather curious omission.

The booklet lists three tips for cutting fat in the diet. They include:

- Cutting down on foods from an "others" category. That fifth catch-all food group includes one dairy food—butter—plus such foods as plain popcorn, cookies, bacon, pretzels, fruit-flavored drinks, potato chips, jelly, and ketchup. Many of those foods actually have low fat levels and some—like plain popcorn—have virtually no fat.
- Limiting fried foods.
- Selecting "a variety of foods within each food group."

That "advice" is insufficient, Contento said. "They ignore the fact that the major source of fat in children's diets is from dairy products," she said.

Only the advice to limit fried foods is helpful in reducing fat. Telling kids to cut down on "other" foods is worthless because the group contains high-fat, low-fat, and non-fat foods. And telling them to eat "a variety of foods within each food group" says absolutely nothing. In the dairy council's view, meaningless generalities are far better than specific, accurate advice that might cause kids to lower their consumption of certain dairy foods.

In all fairness, in recent years the dairy council *has* been modifying its school materials to downplay reliance on the old Basic Four and to tone down their wholesale promotion of dairy foods. Many dairy producers are angry about the changes, Contento said. "My impression is that they don't see the point to all this nutrition education in schools, because it isn't pushing milk enough," she said. Contento added that the backlash is causing state dairy council offices nationwide to reduce their nutrition education efforts.

We wanted to talk to the National Dairy Council about these issues. Despite repeated calls over several months, however, the council could not arrange an interview.

Some companies disguise their true intent by creating innocuous-sounding materials. Oscar Mayer does this with its "Making Food Safe" program for third- through fifth-graders. Who could oppose a program that promotes food safety? Anyone can who glances through the teacher's guide. Teaching kids safe food habits is only one of the program's goals. The other three are to teach kids "that all food is made of chemicals," about "the role of processing in our food supply," and about "packaging and transportation." In plain language, the program indoctrinates students in the glories of highly processed, chemical-filled foods. Those just happen to be the kinds of foods that Oscar Mayer makes. Throughout the program, there's nary a word about the benefits of eating fresh foods.

One activity briefly discusses fat. "Fats supply essential fatty acids," it says, "help the body use other nutrients, and supply energy." That's it. There's no mention that too much fat clogs arteries. Could that be because many of the hot dogs and other products produced by Oscar Mayer are loaded with fat?

Food companies like Hunt-Wesson and Oscar Mayer don't have much incentive to update their school materials. In any

Is It Education or Propaganda?

WITH CORPORATE-sponsored teaching materials flooding classrooms, teachers and parents need to evaluate them carefully to see if they're really educational or are just dressed-up advertising. Here are a few of the questions to ask.

We've adapted some of them from "A Guide For Evaluating Industry-Sponsored Educational Materials," published by the National Association for Industry-Education Cooperation, and from "Choose Well, Be Well," developed by the California State Department of Education.

1. Do the materials help further the curriculum's objectives?

2. Does the material introduce experiences that would not otherwise be available to the classroom?

3. Is the material up-to-date?

4. Does the material deal with controversial issues in a fair way?

5. Does the material present alternative views?

6. Do the materials leave out critical information? For example, does a lesson on vegetable oil leave out the fact that oil is 100 percent fat and that fat should be limited in the diet?

7. Does the material promote a commercial product, service, or idea in a way that would mislead students?

8. Is a brand name or logo overtly displayed in the material?

9. When you cover up any logos on the materials, can you still tell who produced them?

10. Does the learning value of the material outweigh the commercial sales pitch?

update, many of their products would look really bad. An Oscar Mayer beef hot dog, for example, has 13 grams of fat and 460 milligrams of sodium. If Oscar Mayer accurately explained what those numbers mean, some kids might stop eating hot dogs. For the food companies, it's far better to keep sending out their old school materials.

When all the arguments over the materials' quality and the companies' motives are done, one question remains: Do teachers actually use this stuff? They must. If they didn't, companies wouldn't spend the money it costs to produce the materials.

Some teachers eagerly accept materials from food companies and producer groups. "Anyone who will hand out things generally is on the open side, and they have a product that they have decided makes a difference," said Sandra McNellis, a teacher at Shakopee Senior High School in Minnesota and chair of the education section of the American Home Economics Association.

Other teachers are more cautious. "Some things are so blatant," said Marilyn Burdwell, who teaches home economics at Fairmont Junior High School in Boise, Idaho. When Burdwell uses a corporate program, she explains its source to her students. This leads to a discussion about how to evaluate various forms of advertising. Her ultimate goal: teaching kids to be intelligent consumers.

"These are not bad people," Burdwell said of food companies that produce the materials. "They're business people, and they want to meet your needs. But you have to be intelligent about this also."

Alex Molnar, a professor in the Department of Curriculum and Instruction at the University of Wisconsin–Milwaukee, sees the bombardment of teachers with industry-produced materials as a serious problem. Molnar said, "By their sheer volume, sponsored materials threaten to turn the school curriculum into a booming, buzzing confusion. The energy and focus of a school is diverted from the education of children to the promotion of special interests."

Unfortunately, not many teachers have the time, energy, and expertise to judge corporate packages that arrive in the mail. Many, grateful for free or cheap materials to supplement the often meager resources supplied by their districts, use the materials without evaluating them closely.

"The assumption always is that it's up to the teacher to choose and critique the materials," said Joan Gussow, a Columbia Teachers College professor. "That's assuming a great deal of knowledge, sophistication, interest, time, et cetera, on the part of teachers."

Other Corporate Tactics

Providing instructional materials is only one way that food companies and producer groups invade schools. Here are some others:

• **Flooding schools with product samples.** The marketers aim to snare consumers early. When General Mills introduced Fruit Roll-Ups, it arranged for preschool teachers to hand out more than a million samples.[10]

Sending samples to home economics teachers is a particularly effective way of hooking kids. *Food & Beverage Marketing* magazine surveyed nearly 1,000 high school home economics students nationwide. Nearly 70 percent said that if they used a brand-name product in class, they'd be more likely to buy it at the store. The magazine concluded: "A few dollars in freebies to the nation's home-ec classes, apparently, could do wonders for product movement on the supermarket shelves."[11]

• **Advertising on *Channel One*.** Food companies are big advertisers on *Channel One*, Whittle Communications' daily broadcast to high schools and junior highs that includes ten minutes of mostly superficial news and two minutes of slickly produced commercials.

By early 1994, Whittle claimed that 12,000 schools with more than 8 million students received *Channel One*.[12] Schools that sign up get free use of about $50,000 in video equipment, including TV sets, VCRs, and a satellite dish. In return, schools promise that at least 90 percent of their students will watch the whole broadcast, including commercials, every day. That kind of captive audience allows Whittle to charge advertisers staggering rates—reportedly $157,000 per showing of an average 30-second commercial.[13]

The high rates don't deter major food companies, who are forever seeking new ways to reach the teenage market. *Channel One* has carried ads for Bubblicious gum, Skittles, Gatorade, Fritos, M&M's, Snickers bars, Burger King, and Chee-tos.

New York has banned *Channel One* from the public schools. Other states, including California, have vigorously opposed it. And most major educational organizations, including the National Education Association and the National Association of Secondary School Principals, have come out strongly against it.

"The classroom and the curriculum are intended to be a marketplace for ideas, not a marketplace for someone's products and services," said Gary Marx, associate executive director of the American Association of School Administrators. "We simply cannot tolerate the exploitation of students who are a captive audience in the classroom."

Marx said other broadcasters, including the Discovery Channel and CNN, now provide high-quality, commercial-free programs for classrooms. "You don't have to sell the kids to get quality video material," he said. However, in all fairness *Channel One* is the only broadcaster so far to provide schools with the free use of video equipment.

• **Sponsoring label-collection projects.** A growing number of food companies are asking schools to pressure students to eat their products. In January 1990, Procter & Gamble offered elementary schools money for Jif peanut butter labels collected by their students. The company gave schools a dime for each pound of Jif. Procter & Gamble blanketed the nation with magazine ads proclaiming: "The more you buy, the more we'll give to America's schools." Nearly one-third of the nation's elementary schools signed up to participate, according to Consumers Union.[14]

Campbell Soup sponsored a similar program. It gave schools a variety of equipment in exchange for Campbell labels.[15] A Kool-Aid program urged kids to save proof-of-purchase seals to earn computer equipment for their schools.[16]

Molnar, the University of Wisconsin professor, said, "The true cost of these 'free' schemes would be apparent if the loss of student learning time and the cost of staff time needed to administer them was added up."

• **Donating goods or equipment in exchange for getting a product into schools.** This is the most crass *quid pro quo,* a direct trade of student health for equipment. Soft-drink companies are particularly fond of these deals. Pepsi, for example, will give an electronic scoreboard or free Pepsi for an "alcohol-free" prom night if a school will install a Pepsi vending machine. Coke also offers scoreboards in exchange for the right to install a vending machine. In some cases, Coke and Pepsi agree to give schools a percentage of their profits.[17]

It may be too much to expect food companies and producer groups to stop promoting their products via samples, advertising, and exchanges, let alone to publish materials describing the dangers of eating the foods they sell. But if they won't produce complete, accurate publications, schools shouldn't use the materials. Especially not when several respected organizations—including the American Health Foundation and the American

Cancer Society—are producing lively, up-to-date, factual nutrition materials for classroom use.

Nutrition Programs That Work

The best nutrition education programs go way beyond the Basic Four and even the Food Guide Pyramid to teach students how to make healthy choices when selecting foods. They also teach kids how to fight pressures from peers, advertisers, and others to eat bad foods. The ultimate goal: modifying how and what students eat.

Researchers are now studying the effectiveness of the new nutrition education programs. Early results are mixed, but indicate the programs have at least a modest impact on actually changing what kids eat.

A study of the "Know Your Body" program, a five-year curriculum that runs from fourth through eighth grades, found that children who participated ate less fat and more carbohydrates than students in other schools that did not participate in the program. "Know Your Body," developed by the American Health Foundation, includes units on diet, physical activity, and smoking prevention.

The broadest-based nutrition education programs are the most successful. Simply having a teacher stand before a class and give a few nutrition lectures will accomplish little. To change eating habits, the program must target the entire school—from classroom to cafeteria—as well as parents.

A program called "FRESH" was tested by Johns Hopkins Medical School staff. The researchers, working with 12 schools in Baltimore, introduced a battery of parent and teacher workshops, newsletters, health fairs, lessons, and other activities designed to promote heart-healthy lifestyles. After two years of effort, third- and fourth-graders' consumption of fatty and salty foods declined by about 15 percent. The children's blood-cholesterol levels declined by about 8 percent, and their blood pressure declined by about 5 percent.[18]

Another interesting program is "Sembrar y Crecer: To Sow & Grow," developed by Growing Connections, a non-profit group in Tucson, Arizona. The program revolves around a large garden that elementary school students plant and then care for. Teachers use the garden as the jumping off point for weekly nutrition lessons, which are integrated throughout the curriculum, so food issues may come up during science, math, social studies, reading, writing, or art lessons.

Through caring for the garden, students also learn they need to take care of themselves, said Linda Ruth Herzog, executive director of Growing Connections. "The real transference that happens is a child will see that if you water the plants, if you weed them and thin them, if you provide enough sunlight, and if you harvest them when they're ready, then they're going to flourish and do very well," said Herzog. "But if you forget to water them or you don't provide enough sun, they don't do well.

"Children understand that the same thing can happen to their bodies. They make that connection. And they also see the connection between that and taking care of the earth."

One October, a third-grade class in the program voted on the treats it wanted for a Halloween party. To the teacher's shock, the kids passed up candy for vegetables, dip, cheese, and crackers. Their favorite vegetables: radishes and broccoli. "There's the statement that kids like sweets, and they don't like fresh fruits and vegetables," Herzog said. "We've found that isn't true. They just have to be exposed to them."

According to researchers from the University of Arizona, "children [in the program] decreased their consumption of foods high in fat, sugar, and salt by 10 percent through the year they were involved in the program. And children who were in the control schools increased their consumption of those same foods during the same period by 12 percent."

The Pawtucket Heart Health Program in Rhode Island has developed a simpler project for junior high and high school home economics classes. Its "Heart Healthy Cook-offs" teach students the basics of nutrition, how to purchase food, and how to modify recipes to make them healthier.

After learning about guidelines for a healthy diet, student teams select recipes. They modify the recipes to lower fat, saturated fat, sodium, and cholesterol levels. For example, they might replace Cheddar cheese with part-skim mozzarella. Then they analyze the original and modified recipes using a computer and nutrition software.

Finally, they cook the dish and discuss it before a panel of judges that can include the superintendent, principal, or teachers. The judges assess the food's taste and nutritional value, in addition to the quality of the students' presentation.

The cook-off is popular with both students and teachers. "They sensitize their thinking about fat and sodium in the diet, and they really have fun," said Dr. Richard Carleton, principal investigator for the Pawtucket Heart Health Program and professor of medicine at Brown University. Preliminary evidence indicates that some students who participate change their diets enough that their cholesterol levels fall.[19]

There's one key question for any program like FRESH, "Know Your Body," "To Sow & Grow," or the Heart Healthy Cook-off: Will changes in eating habits caused by the program persist into adulthood? No one knows the answer. It will take researchers years to determine the long-term impact of today's new nutrition education programs. Scientific studies aside, though, common sense says that children who develop good eating habits are likelier to have healthy diets in adulthood than kids who weren't taught about nutrition. The good habits will

For More Information . . .

Interested in learning more about successful nutrition programs? The following organizations have developed curricula or materials suitable for use in schools.

To learn more about "To Sow & Grow," you can write to:

Growing Connections
2123 E. Grant Road
Tucson, AZ 85719
(602) 325-7909

A Heart Healthy Cook-off kit costs $20. It includes a manual with lessons for teachers, cook-off instructions, and a list of places where teachers can buy computer software for analyzing recipes. You can order a kit from:

Dr. Richard Carleton
Division of Health Education
Memorial Hospital of
  Rhode Island
Pawtucket, RI 02860

The American Health Foundation has developed two health curricula: "Juno's Journeys: Adventures in Health" for grades K-3 and "Know Your Body" for grades 4–8. Write or call:

American Health Foundation
320 East 43rd Street
New York, NY 10017
(212) 953-1900

The American Cancer Society offers "Changing the Course," a health curriculum for elementary schools. Contact your local chapter or write to:

American Cancer Society
1599 Clifton Road
Atlanta, GA 30329
800-227-2345
(404) 320-3333

The American Heart Association has produced a number of materials suitable for use in schools. You can get copies by contacting your local chapter or by writing to:

American Heart Association
7320 Greenville Avenue
Dallas, TX 75231
(214) 373-6300

become particularly ingrained if parents reinforce at home what their children learn at school.

Regardless of long-term impact, the short-term benefits of strong nutrition education programs are obvious. The best programs are opening children's eyes to food, causing them to think about what they eat, and persuading some to change their eating habits at least temporarily. Those are huge strides in and of themselves. After all, any program like To Sow & Grow that can persuade children to choose vegetables over candy at Halloween must be doing something right.

Schools have a tremendous potential to help students develop healthy eating habits. They can ensure that every student has the opportunity to eat breakfast; that tasty, nutritious foods are available for lunch; and that students receive sound nutrition education in the classroom. By taking those actions, schools send a strong message that healthful eating is important.

Schools send the opposite message if they just serve greasy junk food for lunch, if they let the student council or others sell soft drinks and junk food, if they fail to give teachers the resources necessary to provide strong nutrition education, or if they trade instructional time for *Channel One*'s video equipment. Besides telling students that nutrition is unimportant, many of those actions also give students a clear message that they and their school can be "bought" for the right price.

The underlying problem is that schools receive inadequate public funding. Food companies and other firms are all too happy to help fill this gap. If the school cafeteria is losing money at lunch, Pizza Hut leaps in to save the day. If schools lack the funds for sound nutrition education materials, companies flood them with self-serving propaganda.

This funding gap puts great pressure on schools to give in to commercial influences. There aren't any signs that schools' financial problems will lessen in coming years. Thus, the fight to keep them untainted by commercial pressures will surely heat up.

"As funding becomes tighter, there's certainly the possibility that more entrepreneurs will view schools as a prime market," said Lew Armistead, a spokesman for the National Association of Secondary School Principals. "Schools are going to have to decide as a community how they're going to deal with it."

PART 3

What to Do About Your Child's Diet

CHAPTER 10

Getting Kids to Eat Healthy Foods

When Robbie Votaw was 2½, he decided he didn't like vegetables anymore. In many households, such fussiness would unleash a full-scale war of wills between parents and toddler, with the parents cajoling, threatening, or begging their son.

Not at Robbie's house in Oak Grove, Missouri. His mother, Leslie, devised a simple solution. "I told him that his green beans were Ninja Turtle eggs," she said. "Because I associated it with the Ninja Turtles, who he thinks are just 'it,' he would eat them. I did the same thing with peas. He got excited about them because somehow in his mind he was able to relate them with these characters."

Telling a little fib to get her son to eat vegetables doesn't bother Leslie. "I think he realizes it's like a game, more than an actual deception," she said. "There's nothing wrong with making eating a game if it's put in a positive way."

For generations, parents have used every game, gimmick, and trick imaginable to get their kids to eat healthful foods.

Helping children develop an appreciation of food—what it tastes like, how it's grown, where it comes from, how to prepare it, and how it nourishes the body—is one of the hardest jobs in parenting. It's also one of the most rewarding, as it opens kids' eyes to one of life's greatest pleasures. And with the growing evidence that many diet-related diseases start in childhood, helping children understand what food does to their bodies can help them live long and healthy lives.

So how do you get kids to enjoy—not just tolerate—health-promoting foods? This chapter will tell you. We've collected tips from parents, nutritionists, and doctors from around the country, and added some of our own. We offer these tips with the knowledge that not every tip will be suitable for every family. Use those you like, modify those that have possibilities, and discard the rest.

Every tip springs from our Five Commandments for Raising Healthy Eaters:

1. Relax. You don't have to run a nutrition analysis of every bite your children eat. As long as their diets are basically healthy, eating a Big Mac once in a while won't do any harm.

2. Retain authority over food in your house. You should control what foods are available in your home and what your kids eat when they dine out with you. Don't let those lines of authority become blurred.

3. Before tackling your child's diet, examine your own. Children learn by example. It's virtually impossible to teach children good eating habits if you eat poorly yourself.

4. Start teaching healthful eating habits as early as possible. It's easiest to teach good eating habits if you start when your child is an infant. It gets progressively harder as kids get older.

5. Make mealtimes happy occasions. Eating meals—especially with the whole family—should be one of your child's most enjoyable activities. If your dining-room table becomes a battleground, everybody loses.

You can't go wrong if you remember those five commandments. Although following them won't guarantee that your children will eat healthful diets when they move out on their own, it will provide a framework to ensure that you give them the best start in life possible. After that, all you can do is hope your good influence rubs off.

The First Two Years of Life

The first two years of your child's life can be both the easiest and the hardest years for feeding. They can be the easiest because the child has a limited diet and there's no need to limit fat or cholesterol. They can be the hardest not only because parenthood may be a new and frantic experience, but also because the child is developing so quickly that his or her food desires vary dramatically, even from day to day.

Before we give specific feeding advice, one caveat is necessary: You should always consult your pediatrician when deciding how to feed your infant. Babies vary, and your pediatrician is the best authority to help you design a feeding plan that's correct for your child. With that said, we must add that no pediatrician is God. If the pediatrician's feeding advice doesn't make sense to you, try talking about it. If you're still dissatisfied, find a new doctor.

The first feeding decision is whether to give your baby breast milk or formula. Although formulas have greatly improved over the years, "human milk is the food of choice for infants," said *The Surgeon General's Report on Nutrition and Health.* "It provides appropriate amounts of energy and nutrients, it contains factors that provide protection against infections, and it rarely causes allergic responses."[1] Breast-feeding also fosters bonding between mother and child. Thus, while breast milk and formulas are similar—though not identical—nutritionally, there are reasons beyond nutrition to breast-feed a baby.

For a working mother, breast-feeding may be inconvenient at best and impossible at worst. Many mothers express their own breast milk and store it in the refrigerator. A babysitter can then feed it to the child. Renting a good electric breast pump makes this nuisance easier.

Women who adopt a baby almost always use infant formula. A few, though, are able to produce enough of their own milk to at least partially feed their baby. If you are planning to adopt a baby, you may want to contact the local chapter of La Leche League to learn more about the process called relactation (or any other aspect of breast-feeding).

Full-term babies born to well-nourished mothers usually get all the vitamins they need from breast milk. Some breast-fed babies, though, need supplements of vitamins D and K. Supplements usually aren't necessary for formula-fed babies—as long as parents prepare the formula correctly.[2]

For the first four to six months of life, breast milk or formula is all a baby needs. As recently as a generation ago, doctors said babies should get their first solid food at six weeks of age or even sooner. They changed that advice after new research found that babies' digestive systems can't handle solids and that feeding solid foods too early—before the fourth to sixth month—can lead to overfeeding and food allergies. Also, doctors found that contrary to common belief, feeding babies solids doesn't increase their likelihood of sleeping through the night.[3]

Babies shouldn't drink cow's milk until they're at least 1 year old. While their bodies tolerate breast milk just fine, babies can't properly digest cow's milk. In some infants, cow's milk fed too early can cause bleeding in their gastrointestinal tracts, leading to iron deficiency.[4]

Moreover, there's growing evidence that drinking cow's milk before the age of 1 can increase the risk of childhood-onset diabetes. That's due to the fact that a segment of a protein in cow's milk is identical to a protein on the insulin-producing cells in the pancreas. When children with a particular gene ingest the cow's milk protein, it triggers an immune response. But the immune system, instead of attacking only the milk protein, also attacks the insulin-producing cells. Over time the cells are destroyed, and the child becomes diabetic.[5]

The link between cow's milk in infancy and diabetes is still unproven. But for cautious parents, the evidence is strong enough that they should consider a soy-based rather than a milk-based formula, if they're not breast-feeding.

Some parents, eager to give their babies a good start nutritionally, give them a bottle filled with fruit juice at the first opportunity. That sounds like a good idea, but it's not. Babies shouldn't get fruit juice until they can handle a cup, according to the American Academy of Pediatrics (AAP) and other authorities.[6] The reason: If a baby sucks on a bottle of juice, the juice's natural sugars and acids can remain in the mouth for a long time and attack newly erupting teeth. For the same reason, you shouldn't put a baby to bed with a bottle of formula, milk, or anything else other than water.

Introducing Solid Food

For the first solid food, the AAP suggests a single-grain infant cereal. Rice cereal is non-allergenic and particularly easy to digest, although oatmeal and barley cereals are also good choices. Avoid wheat cereal for a few months because some babies are allergic to wheat and it's slightly harder to digest.

You should introduce solid foods one at a time and not offer more than one new food each week, according to the AAP. That allows you to see if your baby has any food allergies. Some of the foods that most commonly cause allergic reactions are wheat products, cow's milk, egg whites, shrimp and other seafood, and soy products. The weekly interval between new foods also gives the baby time to get used to each food.

Deciding whether to feed your baby strained foods cooked at home or commercial baby food is more a matter of personal preference than anything else. With homemade foods, you know exactly what you're giving your baby. However, commercial baby foods aren't the nutritional disasters they used to be.

Until recent years, commercial baby-food producers dumped salt, sodium nitrite, sugar, and MSG (monosodium glutamate) into their products. Manufacturers did so primarily because parents often taste a food before feeding it to their baby, and the additives made the foods taste better to parents. Babies didn't know the difference, since their palates are quite simple.

Manufacturers have dropped several of the questionable additives after the National Academy of Sciences, American Academy of Pediatrics, consumer groups, and parents protested. Today, you can tell exactly what's in commercial baby food by checking the label on each jar. One additive to avoid is modified food starch, a filler that is not dangerous, but that replaces wholesome fruit or vegetable ingredients.

If you're concerned about pesticides, you can buy organic baby foods. Organic products are made from grains, fruits, vegetables, and other ingredients that have not been treated with pesticides. They also do not contain artificial preservatives, flavors, or colors, and don't have added sugars, salts, or starches.

Whether you feed your child commercial or homemade baby foods, make sure the infant continues to get lots of breast milk or formula. For at least the first year of life, breast milk or formula should provide most of the baby's vitamins and minerals, and solid foods should play a supplementary role.

When you start giving your child cow's milk, stick with 2

percent or whole milk until the child's second birthday. One percent and skim milk don't provide enough calories and fat.

After all we've written about the dangers of fat in the diet, it may seem contradictory to recommend giving an infant whole milk. It's not. All medical authorities who recommend lowering fat in the diet—including the American Heart Association—say parents shouldn't worry about fat until their child is 2. Growing infants need calorie-dense fat for proper growth and development, particularly brain development. Breast milk and whole milk both get about half their calories from fat. A few parents who have severely restricted fat too early have caused growth problems in their infants.

When introducing new foods, you should remember that some small, hard, or sticky foods can cause choking in small children. Such foods include raisins, hot dogs, grapes, popcorn, raw carrots, peas, corn, apple chunks, nuts, hard candy, and peanut butter. You can still serve your child some of those foods, but you should cut them into small pieces or cook and mash them. To further guard against choking, make sure your baby is always sitting upright when eating. Also, be sure to watch children while they eat. By about age 4, children have enough teeth that choking is less of a concern.

Don't be startled if your child's eating patterns shift wildly during his or her first two years. At about the first birthday, a child who previously gobbled everything in sight may suddenly become picky. One reason is that the child's food requirements have dramatically declined relative to his or her weight. During the first year, an infant typically triples his or her birth weight and grows in length by 50 percent. All that growth requires a lot of food. The rate of growth slows in the second year, so the child doesn't need to eat as much.

As if shifting food requirements weren't bad enough, infants also can develop food jags. Jags are guaranteed to drive you crazy, but they're usually harmless. Children on jags will eat

How to Read a Food Label

There's good news about food labels: Most of them have just gotten more useful.

During the 1980s, only about half of all processed foods had any nutrition information at all. Labels were so inadequate that in 1989, then-FDA Commissioner Frank Young admitted in The Washington Post they were "almost unintelligible."

A new federal law, the Nutrition Labeling and Education Act of 1990, requires detailed nutrition labeling on almost all packaged foods. The rules also set strict guidelines for making health and nutrition claims on packages. The U.S. Department of Agriculture, which regulates labels on meat, poultry, and frozen dinners or pizzas that contain meat, has ordered similar label rules.

The new labels (of which there is an example at right) make it a lot easier to select healthy foods for your children. But read carefully: Labels provide nutrition information for a "serving" of the food. Check the serving size to see if it's really the amount of food your child would eat at a meal. If it isn't, adjust all the nutrition information accordingly.

The four most important areas you need to check on every label are the listings for fat, sodium, sugar, and ingredients.

• **Fat:** Labels list the amount of total fat in grams, as well as the "% Daily Value." The Daily Value is the maximum amount of fat one should eat in a 2,000-calorie diet. Remember that over the course of a day children above age 2 should get 30 percent or less of their calories from fat. You can use the chart on page 22 to help determine a sensible fat limit for your child. For instance, children between the ages of 4 and 6 should get no more than 60 grams of fat a day.

The new labels list saturated fat, as well as total fat. It's particularly important to limit your child's intake of saturated fat, which goes straight for the arteries. Use the chart on page 22 to determine your child's daily limit for saturated fat.

• **Sodium:** Labels list the amount of sodium per serving and the percentage of the Daily Value of sodium that a serving of the food provides. Anyone above age 2 should eat a maximum of 2,400 milligrams of sodium daily, and eating 1,800 milligrams is better. To put that in context, half a can of cheese ravioli has 990 milligrams of sodium.

• **Sugar:** Labels list sugar levels in grams. You can convert that to teaspoons, if you want, by dividing by 4. On page 241, there is a chart that can help you determine how much sugar a cereal contains. The government does not recommend a Daily Value for sugar. Note that the sugar listing includes both natural and added sugars.

• **Ingredient list:** Labels list ingredients in descending order of predominance, or weight. If the first ingredients are sugar, fat, water, or white flour, the food probably isn't very healthful. For example, three of the first four ingredients in Lucky Charms cereal are marshmallow bits, sugar, and corn syrup, making it clear that Lucky Charms doesn't belong on

the breakfast table.

Also, check the ingredient list for additives. While some pose no threat (and some—vitamins and minerals—are positively nutritious), avoid those on our "10 Worst" list (see page 66).

Nutrition Facts

Serving Size 1 cup (228g)
Servings Per Container 2

Amount Per Serving

Calories 260 Calories from Fat 120

	% Daily Value*
Total Fat 13g	**20%**
Saturated Fat 5g	**25%**
Cholesterol 30mg	**10%**
Sodium 660mg	**28%**
Total Carbohydrate 31g	**10%**
Dietary Fiber 0g	**0%**
Sugars 5g	
Protein 5g	

Vitamin A 4%	•	Vitamin C 2%
Calcium 15%	•	Iron 4%

*Percent Daily Values are based on a 2,000 calorie diet. Your daily values may be higher or lower depending on your calorie needs:

		Calories:	2,000	2,500
Total Fat	Less than		65g	80g
Sat Fat	Less than		20g	25g
Cholesterol	Less than		300mg	300mg
Sodium	Less than		2,400mg	2,400mg
Total Carbohydrate			300g	375g
Dietary Fiber			25g	30g

Calories per gram:
Fat 9 • Carbohydrate 4 • Protein 4

only a few foods, or maybe only one. Jags aren't harmful if they only last a few days and if the rest of the child's diet is adequate. Instead of being concerned about what your child eats in a single day, monitor his or her diet over a four- to seven-day period. If your child eats a sufficiently varied diet over the extended period, everything is fine.

If you're still concerned, have your infant weighed and measured by your pediatrician. The doctor can tell you whether your infant or toddler is growing at a normal rate. That's the ultimate test of whether the child's diet is adequate.

Sometimes what looks like a food jag is actually a striving for independence. Your tot may suddenly eat only milk in a cup, blueberries, cheese, and crackers. Those are all foods that infants or toddlers can pick up and eat themselves, without any assistance from Mom or Dad. Again, those bursts of independence aren't a problem as long as your child eats a decent diet over a four- to seven-day period.

All the growth changes, food jags, and struggles for independence make it important that you watch for—and respect—your infant's signs that she is done eating. When your baby suddenly eats less as the initial growth spurt ends, it's easy for you to keep trying to shovel in food. That's a mistake. It teaches infants to ignore internal body cues that they're full. Later on, continuing to ignore the body cues can lead to obesity.

Also, trying to feed your baby more than he wants creates a power struggle that you're bound to lose. Babies can control very little in their lives. At an early age, though, they learn that they can control what goes into their mouths. You can control the foods offered to your baby, but you can't force him to eat. On some days, your child may eat far less food than you think he needs. Don't worry about it. Offer the foods you think your baby should have, and let the child eat what he wants. The medical literature doesn't contain a single case of a baby who had food available purposefully starving himself to death. When your child is hungry, he will eat.

Encouraging Good Eating Habits in Your Toddler and Child

Now you're through the easy part. From age 2 on, you can play a much greater role in guiding your child's diet and shaping his or her attitudes toward food. Age 2 also is the point when you need to start keeping an eye on her intake of fat, cholesterol, salt, and sugar.

Age 2 is *not* the time when you turn into the Food Police. You can't force-feed your child "good food" starting at age 2 any more than you could when she or he was younger. Likewise, you can't always stop your child from eating food of which you disapprove. If food becomes a battleground, your child might acquire bad eating habits that could last a lifetime. Your job is to encourage and reinforce good habits, not to bludgeon your child into submission and to insist on perfection.

So how do you encourage good eating habits? "The first thing parents need to do is get control over their own behavior," said Dr. Leonard Epstein, a nationally recognized specialist in childhood eating and obesity at the University of Pittsburgh School of Medicine. That's because children learn by example and want to emulate you.

Mallory Beth Kroll, a 6-year-old member of Kids Against Junk Food (see Chapter 11) who lives in New Jersey, put it succinctly: "I would tell parents to set a good example. Your kids will copy you. Don't keep junk food in the house. Save it for special occasions only."

Watching Your Child's Diet

WHEN YOUR CHILD turns 2, you need to start regulating how much fat, cholesterol, and salt he or she eats. That may sound like a bother, but it's relatively simple.

The most important thing you can do is limit the amount of fat in your child's diet to no more than 30 percent of his or her total calorie intake. Limiting fat is the most effective dietary action you can take to lower your child's risk of heart disease, obesity, and possibly cancer.

How does that recommendation translate into day-to-day reality? To illustrate, let's consider a hypothetical 3-year-old named Peter who eats 1,500 calories daily. Under the guidelines, no more than 30 percent of Peter's calories—or 450—should come from fat. A gram of fat has nine calories, so Peter should eat 50 grams or less of fat daily. To put that number in perspective, consider Peter's fast-food meal. His regular cheeseburger has 13 grams of fat, a small order of fries has 12 grams, and an 8-ounce carton of 1 percent milk has 2 grams. The total is 27 grams, or about half the fat Peter should eat all day.

The National Research Council has also recommended that people above age 2 get less than 10 percent—and ideally only 7 or 8 percent—of their calories from saturated fat, the kind of fat that's most prone to clog arteries. Under the recommendations, Peter should consume no more than 105 calories, or about 12 grams, of saturated fat. Going back to Peter's meal, the regular cheeseburger has 5 grams of saturated fat, the small fries have 2.5 grams, and the carton of 1 percent milk has 1.6 grams. The total is about 9 grams, three-quarters of the amount Peter should eat in a day.

If you control your child's saturated fat intake, you're well on the way to controlling his or her cholesterol intake as well. That's because foods high in saturated fat are also high in cholesterol.

Most experts recommend that people above age 2 eat less than 300 milligrams of cholesterol each day. Ideally, though, children should eat no more than 100 milligrams of cholesterol per 1,000 calories in their diets. Thus, with a 1,500-calorie diet

Peter should eat no more than 150 milligrams of cholesterol.

So how does Peter's fast-food meal stack up cholesterol-wise? The cheeseburger has 50 milligrams, the carton of milk has 10 milligrams, and the fries have none. That's a total of 60 milligrams, or about two-fifths of the cholesterol he should eat all day.

The National Research Council recommends that all Americans—including children above 2—limit their sodium intake to 2,400 milligrams daily. A limit of 1,800 milligrams daily would be better, according to the NRC.

Not surprisingly, Peter's meal is relatively high in sodium. The cheeseburger has 710 milligrams, the small order of fries has 110 milligrams, and the milk has 130 milligrams. The total for the meal is 950 milligrams, half of what Peter should eat for the day.

Obviously, Peter's meal isn't great nutritionally, though it's far better than if he had chosen a double cheeseburger, large order of fries, and piece of pie. It provides three-quarters of the saturated fat, half the total fat and sodium, and two-fifths of cholesterol he should

eat in a whole day. Moreover, it contains no fruit, and fried potatoes are the only vegetable.

Does that mean you should never take your child to a fast-food restaurant? No. What it does suggest is that you should help your child order more healthful choices: salads, carrot sticks, a regular hamburger, or a grilled-chicken sandwich. And if your child does eat a cheeseburger, fries, and milk, balance that meal by serving foods that have lower levels of fat, cholesterol, and sodium at other meals. The key is for your child to have a moderate intake of fat, cholesterol, and sodium over an entire day, or even over three to four days.

Once you're on the right track, you can start helping your child develop healthy eating habits. While there's no proof that childhood habits persist into adulthood, common sense indicates that for many children they do. Children learn from their experiences, and that learning stays with them for life.

One aspect of promoting a healthy diet is introducing your child to a wide variety of foods. Just because your child ate acorn squash at age 3 doesn't mean he or she will necessarily eat it for life. But the fact that you *introduced* squash and other foods may make your child more likely to eat squash in particular and new foods in general in later years. This willingness to try a variety of foods is important in developing a healthy diet—and exciting dining experiences. It doesn't matter whether you succeed in teaching your children to love a particular food. What *does* matter is that you teach them to be open to new foods.

Getting kids to try new foods can be tricky. "Parents don't understand that kids are reluctant to try new things," said Leann Birch, a childhood-eating expert at the University of Illinois at Champaign-Urbana. Parents can get frustrated by this reluctance and give up too easily. They may present a food to their child once and, if she rejects it, never try again. Birch thinks that's a mistake.

"With repeated exposure, kids will come to accept lots of things that they initially reject," she said. "If you're willing to hang in there and re-present items to kids, over time they'll come to accept a fair number of those things."

A good rule is to require children to try one bite of any new food. Don't force them to eat more if they dislike the food. Forcing a child who doesn't like Brussels sprouts to eat them anyway will do nothing but disrupt your dinner. It also might cause your child to develop a lifelong hatred of Brussels sprouts. If your children don't like Brussels sprouts, just require them to try one bite each time you serve them. Over time, they may actually develop a liking for Brussels sprouts. And if they don't, well, there are plenty of other great vegetables out there.

This gets trickier if your child doesn't like the main dish you serve. You certainly can't let the child starve. At the same time, you can't turn into a short-order cook. For such occasions, you should always have alternative foods such as bread, canned tuna, and fruit available.

It's important that you not make a big deal out of your child rejecting a food, even if it's a food that you think the child should eat. You have to respect your child's tastes. After all, each of us—no matter what age—has various foods that we dislike. If your child rejects a food, ask in a calm voice what she or he doesn't like about it. It may be the taste, the texture, the color, the fact that it has touched another food on the plate, or something else. Asking your child for specifics does two things. First, it requires your child to go beyond just saying "Yuck!" to a new food. And second, it can help you figure out how to "fix up" the rejected food or select other new foods the child may like better.

One key in getting your child to accept a new food is presenting it properly. Here are some common mistakes guaranteed to cause problems:

- Asking the child, "Would you like to try this new food?" Most kids will respond with one word: "No!" Simply put a bite of the new food on her plate.
- When offering the food, saying, "We eat this food because it's good for us." That's a sure-fire tip-off that the food tastes terrible. Instead, make it clear you eat *all* foods because you enjoy them. It's fine also to tell your child that certain foods will help him grow up to be strong and healthy. But the first selling point for any food has to be enjoyment.
- Having adults and older children at the table make faces or negative comments about a food when you serve it. For a

young child, those reactions will torpedo the new food faster than anything else. If other family members clearly express their dislike of a food, the child will start with a negative impression before even trying it.

• Overwhelming the child with lots of new foods all at once. Introduce new foods one at a time, and serve them along with familiar foods. This lessens the shock for your child.

So what foods should you introduce to your child? Any and all of them. Most Americans eat only a tiny fraction of the wonderful foods that are available. Widen your child's horizons as far as possible. In fact, every time you go shopping, try to find at least one new food, and try a new recipe at least once a month.

Don't limit the child just to foods that you like. If you don't care for squash, for example, serve it anyway and see how the child reacts. And while you're at it, try a bite yourself to see if your tastes have changed.

Also, don't limit your child just to foods that you think he or she will like. Sometimes your child will surprise you. For example, Joan Vasko, a mother in Toledo, Ohio, found that her two children developed tastes for V-8 juice—which was offered as a special treat before dinner or while taking baths—cranberries, and stewed tomatoes while they were still preschoolers. None of those are foods you'd think young children would especially like.

Making Vegetables a Hit with Kids

If you're like most parents, you're probably more nervous about introducing your child to vegetables than any other food. Maybe you remember with horror all the ploys your parents used when you were young. Do pronouncements like, "You're not leaving the table until you eat all your vegetables!" Or, "I'll give you a big dish of ice cream for dessert if you eat your vegetables!" ring a bell?

Those ploys create all kinds of negative attitudes about vegetables. Forcing a child to remain at the table creates a power struggle between parent and child that extends far beyond vegetables. And what good does it do if, after sitting at the table for hours, a child finally gags down some cold Brussels sprouts?

It's even worse to bribe the child to eat his or her vegetables. Bribery tells the child that vegetables must be truly awful, if such measures are necessary. It also establishes vegetables as something you eat as fast as possible to get to the "good stuff."

Threats and bribery may work in the short term, but they can create lifelong aversions to vegetables. They also can create chaotic mealtimes. There's no need for child-rearing to be that difficult. Instead, there are lots of positive steps you can take to increase the chances your child will like at least some vegetables. All the steps are quite simple. Usually, all they require is that you have a positive attitude that you can share with your child. A few also require a little creativity.

• Try perking up vegetables with seasonings other than salt, butter, or cheese. With a little experimenting, you can find a wide range of spices and juices that add new taste sensations and zest. With broccoli, for example, you might want to try lemon juice, pepper, dry mustard, nutmeg, basil, curry, oregano, or garlic. With steamed carrots, try adding parsley, cinnamon, lemon juice, allspice, nutmeg, mint, caraway seeds, dill seeds, ginger, mace, thyme, marjoram, honey, or pepper. If you do use salt, butter, or cheese, try to add as little as possible.

• Serve fresh vegetables whenever possible, with frozen as your backup. Fresh (and some frozen) vegetables taste much better than canned ones, look prettier, and have a better texture. Nothing will turn off a child faster than if you serve mushy, gray lumps that taste more like metal than vegetables.

• When you cook vegetables, cook them lightly. The best methods are blanching, steaming, microwaving, and stir-frying. All preserve both the nutrients and the taste.

• Serve lots of raw vegetables. Many children who don't like cooked carrots, for example, will gobble them down raw. Children especially like raw vegetables with some low-fat dip or dressing. Don't bother asking your kids whether they'd like a vegetable plate, because they'll likely say no. Just put one out and see what happens. Also, kids who hate cooked cabbage frequently love raw cabbage shredded in a salad with pineapple and other goodies. If you're serving raw vegetables to a child under age 4, cut them into small pieces to avoid choking hazards.

• At a meal, serve the vegetables as a first course. Children are hungriest at the beginning of the meal. If you serve all the meal together, your child may fill up on other foods he or she likes better before getting to the vegetables.

• Be creative in using vegetables' naturally vibrant colors to grab your child's eye. For example, adding bits of sweet red pepper to green beans or broccoli around Christmas may spark your child's interest.

• Tell your young child that peas, broccoli, green beans, or Brussels sprouts are foods loved by his or her favorite cartoon or storybook characters.

• Take your children grocery shopping and let them pick whichever fresh vegetable interests them. Or you can choose the type of vegetable and ask them to select the individual pieces. That gives your children some ownership in the vegetable, making them more likely to eat it.

• When your child is old enough, sell vegetables by explaining their health benefits. Describe how broccoli, carrots, and other vegetables are great sources of fiber, vitamins, and minerals. You can admit that eating vegetables won't turn him into Superboy or her into Supergirl, but explain that vegetables contain substances

The VIPs

A select few fruits and vegetables qualify as VIPs, or Very Important Produce. That's because they have the highest levels of vitamins and/or fiber.

Of course, all fresh fruits and vegetables except avocados are low in fat, and most contain loads of fiber, vitamins, minerals, and other health-promoting substances. But the VIP fruits and vegetables stand above the crowd. They're the ones you should serve your child as often as possible. They include:

• **Fruits:** papaya, cantaloupe, strawberries, oranges, tangerines, kiwi, mango, persimmons, apricots, watermelon, raspberries, and grapefruit.

• **Vegetables:** sweet potatoes, carrots, spinach, collard greens, red pepper, kale, dandelion greens, broccoli, Brussels sprouts, and baked potatoes with skin.

that will help strengthen their bodies for the long haul. If you need to brush up your knowledge about the health benefits of vitamins in vegetables, buy *Jane Brody's Good Food Book.* It is superb and includes terrific recipes.

• When your kids watch TV or use the computer, only let them eat "neat" foods like carrots, grapes, and apples that you or they have cut up and put in child-sized containers. Your kids will think you're being a neatness freak. They won't realize that your additional motive is good nutrition.

• Open and rinse a can of pinto, garbanzo, white, or other beans, and offer them as a snack. They're not low in sodium, but they're a great source of fiber, minerals, vitamins, and protein. Kids love them, partly because they're finger foods.

• If your child absolutely won't eat vegetables, puree veggies and add them to soup. Or chop them into tiny, unrecognizable pieces and add them to casseroles, lasagna, spaghetti sauce, or other foods. If you do this artfully, your child will never know the difference.

If you try all those tips, you're almost certain to find some that work with your child. But what if they all fail? What if your child possesses microscopic vision that can identify specks of the hated zucchini in your turkey loaf?

First, don't panic. Keep reintroducing vegetables, keeping in mind that children's acceptance of foods grows with familiarity. Also, try new ways of preparing dreaded vegetables.

Finally, if absolutely everything fails, load up your child with extra servings of fruit. Fruit and vegetables provide many of the same nutrients. Fruit won't make up all the nutrients lost by not eating vegetables, but it will make up some of them, especially vitamins A and C. Even if you resort to that, though, keep reintroducing vegetables. Eventually, even the hardest case will probably develop a taste for at least some of them.

Other Strategies to Promote Healthy Eating

If you introduce your children to a wide variety of foods, particularly fruits and vegetables, you're well on the way to teaching them healthy eating habits. Here are some other things you can do:

Plant a garden. This is one of the best things you can do as a parent. A garden gives your child "ownership" of vegetables you plant. What child can resist biting into a fresh tomato he or she watched grow and turn fire-engine red? Children's sense of ownership is particularly strong if they help plant, cultivate, and harvest the garden. An added advantage is that you can avoid the use of pesticides.

A garden doesn't have to be large. A 10-foot-by-10-foot plot gives you lots of growing space, but keeps the garden an easily manageable size. If you don't have land for a garden, check with your city or county government to see if there's a community plot nearby. Or plant a garden in your home. If you have some large pots and sunny space on a patio, porch, apartment balcony, or in your house, you're all set. You can plant tomatoes, carrots, and lettuce in one-gallon pots. Make sure there's a hole in the pot's bottom. Then put in about an inch of stones to help water drain. Fill the pot with fine, crumbly soil, and plant your seeds or seedlings. You can get one tomato plant, four or five carrots, or two to three lettuce plants in one pot.

You can plant zucchini squash the same way, although you'll need a half-bushel basket or large tub instead of a pot. Plant six to eight seeds a couple inches down in the soil. When the plants pop up, thin them down to just two plants. Otherwise, you'll end up with a zucchini jungle.

Make most of your meals at home. If you want your child to eat a healthy diet, you must cook most of your family's food yourself. There's just no way around that.

Relying on microwave dinners, fast food, and delivered pizzas is all right occasionally. Most convenience foods, though, are high in fat and sodium and deficient in the nutrients your growing child needs. Most noticeably, they usually lack significant portions of fruit and vegetables.

Of course, cooking food from scratch takes more time than picking up the phone and dialing a pizza delivery joint. But it doesn't have to take lots more time, and it is a lot cheaper.

The first step is to change the structure of your meals. For generations, the traditional American meal has centered on the biggest piece of meat the family could afford. The starches, vegetables, and fruits all played minor roles around this star attraction. Today, you need to reverse those roles. Make the starches, vegetables, and fruits the center of the meal. If you serve meat, give it just a supporting role. There's a common misconception that starches such as potatoes, rice, pasta, bread, and dried beans are fattening. They're not.

When you do cook meat or poultry, use methods that lower the fat content. With poultry, for example, always remove the skin. Much of a bird's fat rests in the skin. With other meats, trim off all the visible fat before cooking. Some cooking styles are more healthful than others. Instead of frying meat, poultry, and fish, try broiling, roasting, poaching, or baking. When you roast meat, place it on a rack so the fat can drip away.

Three pieces of kitchen equipment can help you prepare fast, healthy meals: a crock-pot, a wok or large frying pan, and a microwave oven. With a crock-pot, you can prepare easy stews, soups, roasts, and other dishes by putting the ingredients together in the evening, refrigerating overnight, and placing them in the crock-pot in the morning. Dinner will be ready when the family arrives home. Crock-pots are great for keeping low-fat meats tender and juicy. A wok or large frying pan allows you to prepare a wide variety of healthy stir-fried dishes that take only minutes to prepare. And microwave ovens can bake potatoes or cook vegetables in minutes.

Include your child in the cooking. Cooking helps a child learn reading through the recipes and labels, math through measuring ingredients, science through watching ingredients change during cooking, language through learning words associated with cooking, and nutrition through understanding what nutrients are in foods and determining how to combine foods into a healthful meal. Children also develop motor and perceptual skills by working with food and kitchen implements. And finally, cooking contributes to children's social and emotional development. What other activity teaches a child so much?

Obviously, how much a child can do in the kitchen de-

Healthy Cookbooks For Kids

Most cookbooks designed for children are filled with recipes that are loaded with fat and sugar. The following two books offer child-friendly recipes that promote health.

• *American Heart Association's Kids' Cookbook: All Recipes Made by Real Kids in Real Kitchens* (New York: Times Books, 1993), $15. A beautifully produced book with heart-healthy recipes.

• *Kitchen Fun for Kids* (New York: Henry Holt, 1991), $14.95. Fifty tasty and interesting recipes, each accompanied by a cute drawing and nutrition tip.

pends on his or her age. Even a very young child, though, can help set the table, tear apart lettuce for a salad, snap string beans in half, or scrub vegetables. With supervision, older children can measure and mix ingredients, crack eggs, peel fruits and vegetables, slice or grate, beat with an egg beater, and grind with a meat grinder. They also can help clean up the kitchen after cooking.

Older children can cook simple dishes by themselves. Some parents even let older children plan and cook a whole meal. That gives the children a tremendous sense of accomplishment, besides giving them a voice in choosing what they eat. Not incidentally, it also gives the parents a break from kitchen duties.

Take your child to a pick-your-own farm or a farmers' market. Children have not truly lived until they have gorged on juicy, luscious, organically grown strawberries plucked right off plants in a farmer's field. You can find pick-your-own farms in most parts of the country, even near some of the largest cities.

Taking your child to a farm can be a magical experience, especially for a child who has grown up in the city. Most important, children see how food grows. Too many children today think food grows in frozen boxes in the supermarket.

The next-best choice is to take your child to a farmers' market. Farmers markets usually offer a greater array of fresh fruits and vegetables than a single farm. Let your child select some of the produce you buy. That may increase your child's receptiveness when you serve the produce later.

Take your child to the health-food or grocery store. That isn't as crazy as it sounds. If your child is in a good mood and not tired or hungry and if you're not in a hurry, it can be a tremendous learning experience—and lots of fun for both of you. Whether your child is 2 or 12, there's lots to explore in the grocery store.

The key to a successful trip is involving the child. If you just drag him or her along as you race down the aisles, the trip will likely be a miserable experience for both of you. Instead, teach your child as you go and let him or her help as much as possible in your shopping decisions.

Make sure your child eats before leaving home. A well-fed child is less likely to be demanding at the store. And depending on the child's age, let her or him help you compile the grocery list. Even a young child can look in the refrigerator to see how much milk remains in the carton or can run to the pantry to check the supply of paper towels. That helps teach your child the importance of making a shopping list.

Only your child's age limits what you can do together at the store. Even a very young child can point to different colors as you go down the aisles. The produce section is full of bright colors, making it a great place to teach your child colors.

A slightly older child can help you select fruit and vegetables. If you need apples, let your child choose the individual apples you buy. Use this as an opportunity to teach your child how to select produce. If you're a little braver, let your child choose one fruit or vegetable on his or her own. If you like, save this activity

Four Sure-fire Dinners Kids Will Love

If you want a truly easy, kid-pleasing dinner, have a "build-your-own-dinner" night. Following are four variations, although you should be able to come up with others that your family will like. With each suggestion, all you need to add is low-fat milk and some fruit for a complete meal.

Build-your-own-pita-pockets night. Put out whole-wheat pita bread sliced in half, small pieces of sliced turkey breast or low-fat cheese, and a selection of vegetables including lettuce, sliced tomatoes, sliced onions, sliced cucumbers, bean sprouts, and whatever else you like. Spice it up with mustard, cranberry sauce, or salsa.

Build-your-own-baked-potato night. Bake some potatoes, then let your kids top them with whatever they like. Some good toppings include grated part-skim Parmesan or low-fat cheese, plain non-fat yogurt flavored with curry or dill, ratatouille, vegetables sautéed in water or a little oil, canned (without salt) or frozen peas, and salsa.

Build-your-own-chef's-salad night. Put out lettuce, spinach, diced turkey, lean ham, low-fat cheese, boiled egg whites, cucumbers, cherry tomatoes, carrots, and whatever other vegetables your kids like. You might serve some fresh bread with this meal.

Build-your-own-burrito night. Put out cooked ground turkey, cooked kidney or black beans, hot sauce, black olives, rice, torn-up lettuce, diced tomatoes, and warmed flour-tortillas.

All those meals are quick, easy, fun, and nutritious. They involve your children in creating the meal, increasing the chance that they will eat it. Helping your kids select the ingredients for their dinner also gives you a chance to pass along some nutrition information. Even the cleanup is easy—especially if the kids help!

as a reward for the end of the trip. It sure beats rewarding your child with a candy bar from the checkout lane.

With older children, you can help them find foods produced in a country they're learning about in school. Or you can sharpen your children's math skills by having them add up your grocery bill as you go along.

Even fairly young children can start learning how to read labels. You might begin by explaining how to find a cereal's sugar level. Then, let your child choose any cereal that has 6 grams or less of sugar per serving. Likewise, you can teach an older child how to determine the fat level in a frozen dinner. Then, let your child choose any dinner that gets less than 30 percent of its calories from fat. That's 90 calories or less from fat in a 300-calorie product.

Explaining how to read labels teaches your child the basics of nutrition and how to be a good consumer. It also takes some of the pressure off you in responding to her food requests. Instead of having to say "no" when she requests a specific cereal, you can say "yes" to a wide range of cereals. That puts the pressure on your child to find a cereal that meets your criteria.

Read books about food with your child. Hundreds of picture books feature food in a prominent role. There are books about a town where it snows mashed potatoes and peas *(Cloudy With a Chance of Meatballs)*, a goat who doesn't like the foods his parents serve *(Gregory the Terrible Eater)*, and a grandmother who battles the magical Mr. Sugar *(Mr. Sugar Came to Town)*. Reading one of these books (see "Picture Books About Food," page 236) with your child can provide an opening to discuss a wide range of food issues.

Eat together as a family as much as possible. With today's active lifestyles and the ready availability of food out of the house, in many families the family meal has gone the way of the dodo bird. Everybody's running in different directions, grab-

Sandwich Suggestions

*S*andwiches are a quick, easy meal that kids love. Here are some ideas for healthy fillings; whenever you can, use whole-grain bread.

- Turkey breast slices or other low-fat luncheon meats with lettuce, tomato, and mustard or low-fat mayonnaise
- Tuna (water packed) with low-fat mayonnaise
- Extra-lean beef hamburger (Healthy Choice) or veggie burger (Harvest Burger or Gardenburger) with tomato, lettuce, and ketchup
- Peanut butter (reduced fat) and sliced banana (or mash the peanut butter and bananas together)

- Pita pocket filled with cucumber, sprouts, tomato, green pepper, mushrooms, or other vegetables with low-fat Thousand Island dressing or mustard; let children pick veggies and assemble
- Warm flour tortilla filled with hot cooked beans and salsa
- Pita bread topped with pizza sauce, sliced or diced vegetables, and sprinkling of parmesan cheese and heated in toaster oven

bing whatever food they can as they fly by.

That's not healthy, nor is it conducive to developing good eating habits. Meals grabbed on the fly are rarely healthful. Usually, they consist of some high-fat, high-sodium prepared food zapped in the microwave or typical fast-food fare.

Gobbling down a meal as fast as possible also cheapens food. Food simply becomes fuel, something we ingest so we can get back to the races. Eating ends up providing little pleasure or enjoyment. Those aren't healthy attitudes to teach children.

Arranging to eat meals together can require concerted efforts to juggle schedules, but it's worth it. Eating meals together can make families stronger. Meals can be times of communication

Picture Books About Food

*T*he following list includes some of our favorite picture books that emphasize food. The list is by no means complete. A children's librarian or good bookstore clerk should be able to help you find lots of other books your child will love.

Alexander's Midnight Snack by Catherine Stock. Alexander the elephant eats his way through the alphabet.

Arthur's Christmas Cookies by Lillian Hoban. Arthur's attempt to bake Christmas cookies as a present for his parents doesn't turn out quite like he expected.

The Berenstain Bears and Too Much Junk Food by Stan and Jan Berenstain. Mama Bear helps the family switch from eating lots of junk food to eating healthy food.

Cloudy with a Chance of Meatballs by Judi Barrett. The story of the town of Chewandswallow, where it rains soup and juice and snows mashed potatoes and green peas.

The Giant Vegetable Garden by Nadine Bernard Westcott. A town intent on winning a prize at the county fair is overrun by giant vegetables.

Good Lemonade by Frank Asch, pictures by Marie Zimmerman. When Hank opens a lemonade stand, he learns that using fancy advertising gimmicks isn't enough to sell lemonade.

Gregory the Terrible Eater by Mitchell Sharmat, pictures by José Aruego and Ariane Dewey. Gregory the goat doesn't want to eat the tin cans, rugs, and shirts his parents fix for his dinner.

How My Parents Learned to Eat by Ina Friedman, pictures by Allen Say. The story of an American sailor and a Japanese woman and their attempts to learn to eat with the utensils of the other culture.

How to Eat a Poem & Other Morsels: Food Poems for Children selected by Rose Agree, pictures by Peggy Wilson. A collection of poems about food by Mother Goose, Maurice Sendak, Lewis Carroll, and Carson McCullers, among others.

How to Make Possum's Honey Bread by Carla Stevens, pictures by Jack Kent. Possum and his friends get together to bake bread. A recipe for Possum's Honey Bread is included at the end.

Little Bear's Thanksgiving by Janice, pictures by Mariana. Little Bear's friends struggle to wake him so he can enjoy a Thanksgiving feast.

The Little Old Man Who Could Not Read by Irma Simonton Black, pictures by Seymour Fleishman. When the little old man's wife goes away for a day, he has many misadventures at the grocery store because he cannot read. He thinks wax paper is spaghetti and that soap flakes are oatmeal.

Little Red Hen by Lyn Calder, pictures by Jeffrey Severn. A retelling of the classic tale, with charming drawings.

Mr. Sugar Came to Town (La visita del Sr. Azucar), adapted by Harriet Rohmer and Cruz Gomez, pictures by Enrique Chagoya. Grandma Lupe, the best cook in the neighborhood, battles the influence of the magical Mr. Sugar.

Muskrat, Muskrat, Eat Your Peas! by Sarah Wilson. An animal family plants a huge garden of peas, but Muskrat will not eat any.

Pickle Creature by Daniel Pinkwater. When Conrad's grandmother sends him to the grocery store, he stumbles across the Pickle Creature.

The Rinky-dink Cafe by Maggie Davis, pictures by John Sandford. An insatiable pig takes over a diner on Thanksgiving Day. Written in charming verse.

Sand Cake by Frank Asch. The bear family goes to the beach, where they bake a cake in the sand.

Stone Soup by Ann McGovern, pictures by Winslow Pinney Pels. A retelling of the classic tale.

Yuck! by James Stevenson. Emma brews up a magic potion that fools two nasty old witches.

where family members talk about their day, tell stories, and laugh together.

Don't use food as a reward. Unfortunately, parents typically use foods that are high in fat, sugar, and calories, like candy, ice cream, pie, and cake, as rewards. The problem with this is that it increases their value in a child's eyes. As Birch, the expert on childhood eating at the University of Illinois, said: "We do a lot of things that teach children to like the very things that we then turn around and tell them are bad for them."

Don't worry too much about obesity unless it runs in your family. "Many parents are concerned, but they don't have to be," said Epstein, the childhood-obesity expert at the University of Pittsburgh School of Medicine. Lots of kids go through relatively brief periods where they're stockier than usual. That's often just part of the growing process.

To determine whether your child has a high risk of becoming obese, Epstein recommends simply looking around you. If you, your spouse, and your other kids are obese, a thin child who starts putting on weight may have a problem. But if other family members are all thin, a child who puts on a few extra pounds will likely outgrow the problem.

If your child has a weight problem, Epstein recommends not changing his or her diet until age 5. Putting a child younger than 5 on any kind of weight-reduction diet can be dangerous, he said. At younger ages, you should help your child get more exercise. Encouraging your child to play outside instead of sitting in front of the tube can do wonders for a weight problem.

Even in treating children over age 5, Epstein emphasizes lots of other actions over cutting calories. "Parents need to realize that if they want their child to be different, they have to start modeling," Epstein said. Good modeling means that the *parents* eat properly and exercise. Epstein also emphasizes removing high-calorie foods from the home, teaching healthy eating habits, and praising the child for exercising and eating healthy foods. None of these actions, he notes, involves cutting calories. Yet all of them can be very effective.

Any dietary changes must include the *whole* family, Epstein added. Some families with both fat and thin members try to cook different foods for the two groups. That doesn't work. Neither does having cookies and ice cream in the house just for the thin people. "A family must adopt a program that everybody in the family can and will follow," Epstein said.

He has little patience for parents who say they can't prevent their child from becoming obese because obesity is genetic. "Parents often use that as an excuse," he said. "Genes don't *cause* obesity; they *predispose* you to obesity." Some parents miss that subtle but important distinction. He emphasizes that both a child's genes and the child's environment have important influences on the child's risk of obesity. Thus, if you know your child has genes that tend toward obesity—in other words, if both parents and any siblings are obese—it's even more important to provide a healthful diet and to encourage exercise.

Avoid overfeeding your child. While you shouldn't be unduly concerned about obesity, you also shouldn't push your child to eat more than she or he wants. "Even well-educated parents have really wrong-headed ideas about how much little children need to eat," said Birch. A 2-year-old may only need two tablespoons of peas, Birch said, but some parents try to coerce him or her into eating half a cup. "That can produce all sorts of problems," she said. Worst of all, it teaches the child to ignore internal cues about when to stop eating, which can lead to obesity.

Keep "bad" foods out of the house. It will be easier for your child to acquire a taste for good foods "if the bad foods aren't there," Epstein said. You have to decide for yourself exactly what constitutes a bad food. In general, bad foods are relatively high in fat, cholesterol, sodium, sugar, or calories and provide

How to Choose a Breakfast Cereal

As you and your child turn down the cereal aisle at the supermarket, dozens of different brightly colored boxes scream for attention. How do you choose a cereal that will be at least reasonably good for your child?

All you need to do is read the labels. First, look at the ingredient list. If sugar is the first ingredient, reject the cereal. A top billing means the cereal contains more sugar than anything else. Also, make sure the cereal is made from a whole grain, such as whole wheat. Corn flakes, usually made with degermed corn flour, are not whole grain. And if the cereal has artificial colors or BHA or BHT preservatives, reject it. Those additives are all suspected of causing allergic reactions, a slightly increased risk of cancer, or other problems.

Next, look at the nutrition label for the number of grams of sugar in a serving. The American Dietetic Association recommends rejecting any cereal that has more than 6 grams of sugar per one-ounce serving. A cereal with 6 grams of sugar per ounce is just over 21 percent sugar. To calculate the sugar content of any cereal, use the chart at right.

The 6-gram-per-ounce guideline is helpful unless the cereal contains raisins, dates, or other dried fruit. Dried fruit is high in sugar, so it can boost a cereal's sugar level even if the manufacturer hasn't added any sugar. The cereals you need to watch out for

few nutrients. Examples include soft drinks, hot dogs, fatty steak, cake, ice cream, and doughnuts.

"It's just going to be easier for the kids if those foods are not around," Epstein said. "If they're around, I know from experience that kids are going to eat them."

When counseling children and their families on eating practices, Epstein doesn't ban junk foods from the diet. Instead, he suggests only letting kids eat them outside the home at special

are those in which the manufacturer just dumped lots of sugar.

Next, check the cereal's fat content. Most cereals have very little fat, but there are exceptions. For example, some granolas have 8 grams of fat in a small one-ounce serving. Getting 8 grams of fat from a breakfast cereal takes a good chunk out of your child's daily fat quota.

You should ignore the big print on the box boasting about all the vitamins the cereal contains. The vitamins aren't bad, but they don't make the sugar and additives go away. Vitamins are added more as a marketing gimmick than anything else.

Grams of sugar per one-ounce serving	Percentage sugar by weight	Teaspoons of sugar per one-ounce serving
2	7	½
4	14	1
6	21	1½
8	28	2
10	35	2½
12	42	3
14	49	3½
16	56	4
18	63	4½

events like birthday parties, ball games, or holiday celebrations. Keeping junk foods out of the house reduces temptation, while letting kids eat them elsewhere provides a little leniency.

Don't worry unduly about what your child eats outside your home. Try as you might, you can't always control what your children eat elsewhere, especially as they get older and have more money in their pockets. Even if you pack a healthful

Selecting the Best Hot Dog

IN A PERFECT WORLD, your child wouldn't like hot dogs or hot dogs would be healthful. But a typical hot dog is a bunch of meat scraps, grease, water, salt, and additives pumped into a skin. Few foods are worse nutritionally.

In the real world, though, most kids love hot dogs. So if you can't see eliminating hot dogs from your child's diet, serve the healthiest hot dogs available. Fortunately, some manufacturers are responding to health concerns by producing lower-fat hot dogs.

How do you find the best hot dogs? Read the label—carefully. Reduced-fat hot dogs often contain 10 or more grams of fat (75 percent of calories), compared to about 16 grams (80 percent of calories) for a regular beef frank. Surprisingly, many hot dogs made from chicken or turkey are little better than their beef counterparts.

Hot dogs also contain lots of sodium. A regular beef hot dog has about 585 milligrams, while a bun has about 240 milligrams and a teaspoon of mustard has 60. Thus, just two regular hot dog sandwiches with mustard provide almost all the sodium a child should eat in an entire day.

Many of the hot dogs touted as healthy alternatives have sodium levels that are even higher than those in all-beef franks. For example, a Butterball Turkey Frank has 610 milligrams of sodium, and an Oscar Mayer Light Wiener has 623 milligrams.

The best hot dogs have no more than 4 grams of fat and 500 milligrams of sodium. Some that meet this standard are listed below. The low-fat hot dogs taste fine, although different from the old-fashioned frank. Adding mustard and other condiments results in a taste almost everyone will enjoy.

HOT DOG	FAT (GRAMS)	SODIUM (MG)
Yves Veggie Cuisine Fat-Free Veggie Wieners	0	249
Lightlife Fat-Free Meatless Smart Dogs	0	290
Healthy Choice Franks	1	460
Yves Veggie Cuisine Tofu Wieners	4	116

lunch for school, your child may trade his or her apple for a Twinkie. And if your child plays at a friend's house, the parents may serve foods that don't meet your nutritional standards.

All you can do is teach good food habits and hope your child remembers them when he or she is out of your sight and control. An occasional slip will do little harm as long as the overall diet is healthy.

If you go to a fast-food restaurant, make healthy choices. A trip to a fast-food restaurant can be a nutritional disaster for your child, but it doesn't have to be. Today, fast food isn't automatically junk food. In the last few years, the fast-food giants have finally realized there's a market for healthier fare. Some of the changes include:

• Wendy's has an excellent salad bar, and Burger King, McDonald's, and other chains offer packaged salads.
• Wendy's and some other chains offer baked potatoes.
• McDonald's has introduced a lower-fat hamburger.
• McDonald's offers non-fat apple bran muffins, carrot sticks, frozen yogurt, 1 percent milk, and Cheerios and Wheaties.

These and other changes make it possible to buy your child a healthful meal at most fast-food restaurants. That's not to say that fast-food restaurants have become health-food emporiums. They haven't. Most of the foods on their menus still contain far too many calories and too much fat, saturated fat, cholesterol, salt, or sugar. But if you choose carefully, you can do quite well.

Unfortunately, the fast-food chains have fought off government efforts to force them to disclose nutritional information. Some chains make nutritional information available, but usually only upon request.

You can get detailed nutritional information by asking a clerk at the fast-food restaurants you patronize for a brochure.

Getting the Best from Fast Food

*H*ere are some general tips on how to choose a healthy fast-food meal for your child:

• **Avoid specially packaged kids' meals.** They're bad values both nutritionally and monetarily. Most contain a burger, fries, and a soft drink. Instead, get your child a grilled chicken, small burger, or other sandwich; a side salad, carrot sticks, or baked potato; and low-fat milk.

• **Stay away from sandwiches called "whopper," "double-decker," or "super."** Most contain lots of unnecessary calories and fat. Small burgers or the lower-fat McLean Deluxe are the best bets if your child wants a burger.

• **Order burgers with as few toppings as possible other than vegetables such as lettuce, tomato, and onions.** Mustard and ketchup are high in salt, but they're a better choice than cheese, bacon, mayonnaise or tartar sauce, which are fatty. Fortunately, some chains are switching to low-fat mayonnaise.

• **Order baked potatoes carefully.** For toppings, choose vegetables only or a pat of margarine. Cheese, butter, and sour cream toppings add lots of fat, changing potatoes from healthy foods into unhealthy ones.

• **Encourage your child to try the salad bar or a packaged salad.** Use a low-calorie dressing.

• **Processed meats have lots of fat and sodium.** Skip pepperoni on pizza and sausage on a biscuit.

• **Remember that fish and chicken aren't necessarily healthy choices.** Many chains bread or batter their fish and chicken and deep-fry them. Then they smear

Or you can write to the company's consumer-affairs director.

Don't rely on vitamin supplements to cure a bad diet. A multi-vitamin supplement or doses of vitamin C does not replace the need to eat a healthy diet. Vegetables and other natural foods contain a wide variety of health-promoting substances

mayonnaise or tartar sauce all over the sandwich. All this jacks up the fat and calorie levels well beyond those of a basic burger. If your child orders a deep-fried food, try to strip off the skin or breading. A better choice is to order baked or broiled chicken or fish, if it's available.

• When ordering a pizza, try one that's cheeseless and topped with tomato sauce and lots of vegetables. That may sound strange, but can be delicious. Alternatively, ask for half the usual amount of cheese. If your child won't go even that far, order a regular, thin-crust pizza with cheese and vegetable toppings instead of a deep-dish pizza with extra cheese and meat toppings.

• At breakfast, steer your child away from the croissant and biscuit sandwiches. Most are full of fat and sodium. Instead, get a bagel or go to McDonald's and get your child Wheaties or Cheerios, low-fat milk, orange juice, and an apple bran muffin. Pancakes are not a bad choice at various restaurants, provided you don't drench them in syrup.

• Instead of visiting a fast-food restaurant, try a grocery store for a quick meal. Many now have extensive salad bars, deli sections, and soups. After helping your child select soup, a sandwich, or salad, pick up some apples, oranges, or bananas, some bagels or whole-wheat pita bread, yogurt, and a carton of juice or low-fat milk. Take your lunch to a park for a picnic. Or bring it home and spread out a blanket on the floor for an at-home picnic. Either type of picnic may be more fun than sitting in a crowded, noisy fast-food restaurant.

not found in supplements. You also don't want to teach your children that "health" comes out of a bottle of pills.

If your child suffers a food-related illness, use it as a learning experience. For example, your child may get sick after eating lots of high-fat, high-sugar foods at Halloween or a party.

Use the opportunity to explain that what we eat affects how we feel day-to-day. A young child may not be able to relate to the idea that eating healthy foods helps prevent heart disease and cancer. But if your child ate too much candy and got an upset stomach, the cause-and-effect relationship between food and health becomes much clearer.

Help your child understand TV commercials for food. If your child watches TV, you can help counteract the influence of commercials. "The single most important thing parents should do regarding television is to watch children's television and the commercials therein *with* their children," said Robert Liebert, an expert on children's television at the State University of New York at Stony Brook.

While watching the commercials, point out to your child the manipulative practices the advertiser uses. For example, explain how fruit always appears in cereal commercials so the manufacturer can claim that the cereal is part of a nutritious breakfast. When a cereal commercial appears, have your child watch for the fruit. How many kinds of fruit can your child spot in cereal ads? How long does the fruit appear on the screen?

Liebert also educates his children about toy commercials. If the commercial makes a toy car look big, Liebert takes his children to a toy store to see how big it really is. Almost inevitably, the car is much smaller than it looked on TV. You can use this same technique with premiums offered in cereal or fast-food commercials. If your child thinks the premium looks great on TV, go to the grocery store or fast-food restaurant and try to find out what it really looks like.

Television reformer Peggy Charren also advocates watching TV with your child, saying, "You can't help counter these messages to your children if you don't know what they're learning."

Charren suggests helping your children develop their own

"commercials" for a food. Through writing ads, your children learn about the manipulative techniques advertisers use. Your children also can write pretend ads spoofing TV commercials for various foods. If you own a camcorder, your children and their friends can act out the ad and watch the results. Charren said that is a terrific activity for birthday parties.

Of course, the best way to counteract TV's influence is to encourage your children to watch public TV or videos that you approve of or to be so busy with other activities—from reading to running—that they don't even want to watch TV. You can designate TV-free nights when your family does something together, preferably something active like skating, walking, or bike riding. Kids should develop active lifestyles starting at an early age. They're unlikely to do so, though, unless you set a good example. If you spend every night plopped in front of the TV, your child will probably do the same.

So what if nothing works with your child? What if, despite your best efforts, your child rejects every remotely healthy food that you serve? Don't panic. You're not as alone as you might think. Even parents of kids you'd expect to be perfect eaters can run into problems.

Take Marion Nestle, a leading nutritionist, who heads the nutrition department at New York University and also was managing editor for *The Surgeon General's Report on Nutrition and Health*. You might expect she never had problems getting her kids to eat healthy food. But you'd be wrong.

When her son was in high school, he wouldn't eat any vegetables. Nestle didn't panic. "I sat down with my son the non-vegetable eater and gave him a nutrition lecture," Nestle said. She did that just once. Then she left him alone. Eventually, he started eating vegetables again.

As Nestle's experience shows, you can't force your child to eat

Dealing with Teenagers

MUCH OF WHAT WE'VE SAID in this chapter is primarily aimed at pre-teens. Teens can be a much tougher nut to crack. Pretending that a spoonful of peas is dinosaur food won't work. On top of that, teens' junk-food habits may be deeply ingrained. Their friends may jeer at anyone who cares about diet and health. And many parents are relieved that their kids are drinking Coke and not wine coolers or beer.

With some kids, simply providing clear information on the benefits of good nutrition and links between diet and disease might be enough to spur better eating habits. Tell your teen about how diets high in fat and salt and low in fiber can promote fatal diseases. If any of your close friends or relatives died of diabetes, colon cancer, a stroke, or heart disease, discuss the dietary connection.

You can also look for role models. Many teens idolize athletes and movie stars, some of whom have foresworn steak-and-egg breakfasts for healthy diets. Have any such people been profiled in newspapers or magazines touting healthy diets and lifestyles?

The teenage years are often a rebellious, anti-establishment period. Some high school kids turn to a more healthful, natural-foods diet to "stick it" to giant food conglomerates—the RJR Nabiscos and ConAgras. Such kids love detecting labeling tricks, or seeing how much air and how little cereal goes into those giant boxes, or discovering that food manufacturers replace real fruit with food dyes and artificial flavors.

Another approach to encour-

a healthy diet. All you can do is set a good example, make healthy foods available, and do everything possible to encourage your child to try them. Then you cross your fingers and hope for the best. Your child, like Nestle's, may occasionally stray. But

age teens to care about nutrition is to link diet to environmentalism. Point out that growing some of your own food, or buying locally grown food at farmers' markets, cuts down on transportation costs and air pollution from gasoline. Buying organically grown foods reduces pesticide and fertilizer use, thereby reducing water pollution. Buying more natural foods and fewer processed foods cuts down on packaging and garbage.

In recent years, more and more teens have seen mankind's raising and slaughtering of livestock as an ethical issue. Who, they ask, gave humans the right to kill other species? Questions like that are often the first step to healthful vegetarian diets. Books like John Robbins' *Diet for a New America* and Frances Moore Lappé's *Diet for a Small Planet* link health with environmental and ethical concerns and have spurred many teens not just to healthier diets, but to social activism on behalf of animals, hungry people, and planet Earth.

Another road to healthy eating habits is to volunteer at a local food co-op. Just being around all those natural foods for a few hours a week is an education in nutrition, agriculture, and the environment. We don't know of anyone whose stint in a co-op didn't improve his or her eating habits. Similarly, volunteering at a soup kitchen or homeless shelter and seeing hunger firsthand puts food in perspective. Knowing how many people are desperate for a nutritious meal makes it hard to chow down on a thick, fatty steak or ten-ounce package of greasy chips.

if you keep at it and don't give up, there's a good chance your child will develop eating habits that will help him or her live a long, healthy life.

CHAPTER 11

What You Can Do Outside Your Home

W hen Beverly Laprade and other parents asked the Pawtucket, Rhode Island, school committee to serve breakfast in the city's poorest schools, they got stonewalled. So Laprade took the next logical step. She ran for the school committee—and she won.

Working from the inside, she got a breakfast program into two of Pawtucket's fifteen schools, and she's confident that Pawtucket will eventually offer breakfast in all of its schools.

Laprade's gumption in running for the school committee puts her in a class by herself. But other parents around the country are working in more modest ways to improve the nutritional environment for children. They're trying to make school lunches more healthful, fast-food meals more nutritious, and TV food commercials more honest.

These parents realize that bad influences outside the home undermine their efforts to raise children with healthy eating habits. That spurs them to get involved in nutrition issues at the local, state, or national levels.

As Laprade and others can testify, such activism is often bruising and frustrating. However, it also is very rewarding—even if you don't win. Knowing that you put up a good fight for children is its own reward, and chances are you've educated a lot of people in the process.

Improving School Food

So what can you do? Everything from simple activities such as writing letters to complex projects such as undertaking a school-breakfast campaign. All have the potential to significantly improve the diets and health of children, yours included. See if any of these ideas fits your interests and talents:

Help your school provide nutrition education. Some parents are working with their local PTA to raise funds for materials that their schools otherwise couldn't afford. While other parents may be pushing for a new roof or computer lab, you should make sure that nutrition films and videos, books, software, and resources get on the list of possible purchases.

A great gift to your elementary or middle school could be a performance of FOODPLAY, a traveling nutrition theater show that features juggling, puppets, music, and audience participation. Barbara Storper, the nutritionist founder of FOODPLAY, also directed the production of one of the best nutrition videos. "Janey Junkfood's Fresh Adventure," which won an Emmy Award as a TV special, uses clever acting, juggling, fancy graphics, and other devices to teach kids about fat, sugar, additives, and label reading. (Call 1-800-FOODPLAY or write to FOODPLAY, 251 Chestnut Ave., Jamaica Plain, MA 02130, for more information. The video costs $99.)

Work to improve the nutritional quality of school lunches. Schools that serve little more than hamburgers, hot dogs, and chicken nuggets hamper your efforts to raise children who eat properly. On the other hand, a strong lunch program that serves nutritious meals can reinforce your efforts at home.

The first step in improving school lunches is assessing their quality. You can get some clues from lunch menus. At a minimum, menus will help you figure out what questions to ask the cafeteria manager or food service director. "I would caution parents from making a judgment by purely reading the menus, since there can be so much variation between products," said Tami Cline, the former assistant director of food services for the Boston Public Schools.

For example, hamburgers can vary widely in their nutritional quality. One school may grill high-fat commodity patties. Another may bake lower-fat patties in perforated pans that let much of the fat drip away. Thus, if the menu lists hamburgers, you should ask how cooks prepare them.

The menu may list many processed foods like chicken nuggets, pizza, or fish patties that suppliers provide ready made. Find out how much fat, cholesterol, and sodium those products contain. Find out, too, whether the district shops among suppliers to find the most healthful, not just the cheapest, version of those foods.

You also can check menus for how often fresh fruits and vegetables appear. Good menus, like those published by the Fairfax County Public Schools in Virginia, even list the fat levels of selected lunch offerings.

You can learn much by inviting yourself for lunch at school, said Vivian Pilant, director of food services for the South Carolina Department of Education. She suggests introducing yourself to the cafeteria manager and asking a few questions. See the sidebar on page 254 for some ideas for questions.

While you're eating lunch, check the cafeteria's serving line.

Are foods attractively displayed? Are vegetables cooked properly so they are moderately crisp rather than soggy? And are foods kept at proper temperatures? Also note whether the servers are pleasant. Food servers' attitudes may seem unimportant, but they're just "as important as the food itself," said Ed Benson, a citizen activist who's chairman of the Nutrition Task Force of the Dade County, Florida, School Board. "If they're forcing kids to take food and rushing them through, then these students aren't going to be happy with anything that comes out of the kitchen." Also check whether students have enough time to eat, and whether the cafeteria itself is reasonably pleasant.

Armed with your knowledge, you're ready to talk to whoever plans the meals. In most districts, that's the food service director. It helps if you can convince other parents—especially leaders of your PTA—to accompany you to the meeting. There's always greater strength in numbers. However, you can go it alone if you wish.

Your first contact with the food service director requires all the tact and diplomacy you can muster. "What tends to happen is people come in and say, 'Your food is awful,'" said Elaine Keaton, food service director for the Albuquerque Public Schools. Not surprisingly, that approach almost always fails. "The director tends to get defensive and say, 'These people don't know what they're talking about,'" Keaton said.

Benson remembers his first approach to food service officials in Dade County. "They were skeptical," he said. "They thought we were there to crucify them." Benson assured them that that wasn't the case. He credits his non-confrontational approach with opening the channels of communication.

"We did not attempt to change things in a week," he said. "We did not tell them all the horrible things they were doing. We said, 'We are here to work with you to try to improve the quality of the food we're feeding our children.'"

Questions to Ask About School Lunch

When you meet with the school food service director, you should indicate how important you believe good nutrition is to children's health. Ask about the director's interest in nutrition and his or her plans for making the lunch period an enjoyable, educational experience. Before meeting with the director, you should know as much as you can about the lunches. Here are some matters to investigate:

1. Are the meals prepared at the school or elsewhere?

2. Does the school contract with an outside firm to prepare lunches? If so, does the school include nutritional requirements in the contract?

3. Is the lunchroom pleasant?

4. Do children have enough time to eat?

5. Do teachers eat with the children?

6. Does the school follow specific nutritional guidelines for fat, saturated fat, sodium, and whole grains when it prepares the lunches? If so, what are they?

7. How much fat and sodium does the average lunch contain?

8. How often are fresh fruit and vegetables served?

9. Is 1 percent milk the standard milk offered?

Always remember that food service directors must operate within constraints. For example, they must cope with budgets, students' likes and dislikes, and free government commodities that are often high in fat and sodium. Those constraints can make compromises necessary.

Benson also cautions that change won't happen overnight. "Anyone who is trying to make changes within this humongous bureaucracy had best understand it's not a three-month or even

10. How often are whole-grain bread and brown rice served?

11. Is there a serve-yourself salad bar?

12. How often are vegetarian entrees offered?

13. How often are fried foods served?

14. Are low-fat or low-sodium versions of hot dogs, cheese, mayonnaise, ice cream, canned vegetables, or soy sauce used?

15. Is any effort made to eliminate the use of questionable additives?

16. Does the school ever try to buy organically grown or pesticide-free food?

17. Do junk-food vending machines and fast-food outlets compete with the standard school lunch for the children's attention?

18. Is the cafeteria seen as an opportunity to teach children about food and nutrition, such as by listing the fat and calorie content of foods, indicating where foods come from, or highlighting the vitamin A and vitamin C content of fruits and vegetables?

19. Are low-income children who receive free or reduced-price lunches in any way made to feel different?

a one-year commitment," he said. "Very little happens in a system in a year."

Sometimes, the food service director won't cooperate with you at all. If that happens, go up the chain of command. Contact the school official who oversees the food service director, the superintendent, or the school board. If you still hit a brick wall, keep recruiting more parents to your cause and contact your local news media. One newspaper or TV story, or a well-written letter to the editor of your local paper, often can do wonders in knocking down roadblocks.

Work to get a state requirement that school lunches be nutritious. This is an especially good idea if you run into a brick wall locally.

You can approach state officials in two different ways. First, you can ask the child-nutrition director in the state department of education to develop nutrition rules limiting the fat and sodium content of meals. Or you can ask state legislators to pass a law requiring that schools serve more nutritious lunches.

"Parents should use every means available to them, working through the local arena first and then working through the state agency or the legislature," said Maria Balakshin, child-nutrition director in the California Department of Education.

The tactics for approaching state government are the same as for approaching local school officials. The first step is to organize other parents. Balakshin said she would respond to an individual parent, "but I would probably take a group of parents or a coalition of parent groups even more seriously." After organizing locally, contact your legislator or an education department official to arrange an appointment. Balakshin advises having a carefully prepared proposal to present at the meeting.

To help develop awareness, invite your local legislator to lunch at school. In 1989, the California Legislature passed a school-nutrition law after a lawmaker visiting a school saw that lunch consisted of corn dogs and tater tots. The law required the state education department to develop voluntary nutrition guidelines for school breakfast and lunch, competitive foods, and child-care food programs. Those guidelines include reductions in fat and sodium and increases in whole grains, beans, and fresh fruits or vegetables. In 1992, 20 pilot school districts and child-care programs were studying how to revise meals, what training workers need, and what the changes will cost. In

1993, another 24 agencies adopted the guidelines. Eventually, Balakshin hopes to release the guidelines statewide.

Balakshin said the law has had "a tremendous impact" that will keep growing. "We hope to have guidelines that will apply not just to the cafeteria but to the total school campus," she said, "and a direction on how to implement these guidelines."

You can ask the legislature or education department in your state to adopt statewide guidelines like California's. Or, if you're ready for a harder fight, you can seek a state law or rule limiting the amount of fat, cholesterol, sodium, and sugar in school lunches. You can accomplish much at the state level. The only limit is how much time you can devote to the fight.

Get vending machines and other sources of "competitive" junk foods removed from your child's school. At many schools, students can buy candy, chips, and soft drinks from vending machines, a student council "store," or fundraising tables run by various student groups. All those temptations encourage kids to eat junk foods instead of the school lunch.

If you try to eliminate those sources of junk foods, expect a tough fight. For starters, you'll be fighting kids who want them. You'll also be battling whoever makes money from them. That may be the school principal, athletic department, student council, or other student groups. Banning junk-food sales could cost whoever profits from them thousands of dollars in lost revenue.

Your biggest ally in the fight will likely be the school food service director. Almost universally, directors hate vending machines and other sources of competitive foods that reduce cafeteria revenue. In working to improve school food, you may want to tackle competitive foods before taking on the cafeteria itself. That way, you'll have built strong lines of communication with the food service director before you try to improve lunch offerings.

Instead of getting rid of competitive foods, it's sometimes much easier to work to improve their nutritional quality or limit

How to Improve School Meals

*M*odifying recipes is one of the cheapest—and easiest—ways to make school lunches more healthful. The following tips are adapted from "The Healthy Edge," a program developed by the School Food Service Foundation. Ask the cafeteria manager how many of these suggestions are being incorporated at your child's school.

TO LOWER FAT, SATURATED FAT, AND CHOLESTEROL:

• Cook with skim milk, part-skim mozzarella cheese, and low-fat yogurt instead of full-fat dairy products.

• Substitute low-fat yogurt or whipped low-fat cottage cheese for sour cream or mayonnaise.

• Make dressings with skim milk or buttermilk instead of mayonnaise, sour cream, etc.

• Avoid seasoning with fat-back or bacon grease.

• Mix ground beef with ground turkey or completely substitute ground turkey for ground beef. (Remember to increase spices by one-fourth to one-third to make up for the milder flavor of turkey.) Drain fat after browning.

• Substitute dry beans for half or more of ground beef in tacos, burritos, or chili.

• Substitute vegetable oils for animal fats.

• Brush the tops of cinnamon rolls with water instead of melted butter before baking.

• Serve only enough gravy or sauce to make a dish acceptable.

• Moisten and sweeten baked goods with dried fruits, fruit juices, or applesauce, and reduce the fat.

• To reduce cholesterol in scratch-baked items, replace some or all of the whole egg with egg whites in equal volume—two egg whites per whole egg.

• Prepare your own dressings to cut down on the amount of oil used, or buy low-fat dressings.

• Prepare cakes and similar desserts from scratch when feasible and reduce the fat, salt, and sugar.

TO INCREASE WHOLE GRAINS BEANS, AND DIETARY FIBER:

• Try replacing at least one-half of the white flour in a recipe with whole-grain flour.

• Use pureed, cooked dried beans, bulgur, or barley to thicken soups.

• Replace some or all of white rice with brown rice.

• Make oat flour by putting oatmeal through the blender. Use it as you would any other flour.

• Combine oatmeal with ground beef for meat loaf, tacos, and similar dishes to increase fiber.

TO MODERATE SUGAR:

• When possible, use less of all sugars, including white, brown, powdered, raw, honey, and syrups.

• Use spices like cinnamon, cloves, nutmeg, allspice, and ginger in recipes when sugar is reduced.

• Replace frosting with powdered sugar or fruit.

• Offer unsweetened fruit sauces for toppings, such as applesauce for pancakes or waffles.

TO REDUCE SALT AND SODIUM:

• Always try using much less salt than recipes call for.

• Use saltless seasoning mixes.

• Use fresh meats in recipes instead of canned ones.

• When fat or salt is reduced, enhance the flavor with bay leaf, basil, parsley, dry mustard, nutmeg, lemon juice, oregano, onion, garlic, pepper, sage, thyme, chili powder, or paprika.

• Try low-salt or salt-free sauces, soup bases, and bouillon or make these items from scratch. Work with one-half low-salt soup base and one-half regular to start.

Finally, suggest that the school food service department buy a copy of *Healthwise Quantity Cooking*, which has dozens of healthy adaptations of standard recipes. It is available for $29.95 from CSPI, 1875 Connecticut Avenue, NW, Suite 300, Washington, DC 20009.

the hours they operate. Vending machines and student stores can sell fruit juices instead of soda pop; low-fat, air-popped popcorn instead of potato chips; and fresh fruit instead of candy.

Push your state to regulate competitive foods. If your district refuses to ban or improve competitive foods, contact state officials. Encourage your state department of education to adopt a rule regulating competitive foods. For example, the state board of education in West Virginia adopted a rule barring schools from selling soft drinks, candy, gum, and ice cream bars during school hours.

If the education department is unresponsive, ask state legislators to pass a competitive-foods law. In Massachusetts, the legislature passed a law forbidding schools to sell soft drinks and candy during the school day.

The West Virginia rule and Massachusetts law are just two examples of what can be done about competitive foods at the state level. Getting such rules or laws passed isn't easy. However, it can be done if you organize parents, educators, and nutrition groups in your state.

Get a School Breakfast Program started in your district if it doesn't have one. This is one of the most important projects you could tackle. Even if you feed your children breakfast every day, there undoubtedly are parents in your district who can't afford breakfast. Their children deserve the same educational opportunity as yours, but don't get it if their stomachs are empty.

Any district that wants to start a breakfast program automatically qualifies for federal funds to help pay for it. For some districts, the federal money pays the entire cost of breakfast. Some districts even make a small profit. Other districts must subsidize their breakfast programs, but the cost is usually minimal.

To help districts pay start-up costs of breakfast programs, the U.S. Department of Agriculture has been providing millions of dollars in grants. Some states, including California, are developing grant programs of their own. Thus, there's lots of start-up money available to districts that seek it.

Often, though, school districts need a little nudge. In Pontiac, Michigan, parents joined with the Hunger Action Coalition for Southeastern Michigan to press for a breakfast program. At first, the group ran into resistance. Most school administrators "weren't all that sold on" breakfast, recalls Joyce McClellan, one of the parents. Despite strong support at a public hearing for a breakfast program, the school board refused to start one, claiming it would cost too much.

The parents and other coalition members kept talking to school administrators. Then they got some key help: The nonprofit Food Research and Action Center included Pontiac in a nationwide hunger survey. The Pontiac results were startling: In poor families, 29 percent of the children under age 12 were hungry (as determined by an eight-question survey). Another 38 percent of the children were in danger of becoming hungry.

Coalition members had worked closely with the news media throughout their campaign, and the media really ate up the survey results. The local newspaper started running editorials criticizing the school board for turning down breakfast when so many children were hungry.

Eventually, the school board agreed to start a breakfast program in the two neediest elementary schools. Lily Webb, another parent, thinks the coalition just wore down the board. "I think they got tired of listening to the facts and decided to give the program a try," she said.

The survey was the key factor in getting breakfast approved, according to Shirley Powell, executive director of the Hunger Action Coalition. Parents' persistence also was instrumental, she said. "Whenever it becomes less hassle to have a program than not to, districts will implement it," she said.

Teachers love the breakfast program, Powell said. "They've definitely seen a decrease with tardiness and absenteeism," she

said, "and children are more attentive." And district officials report the breakfast program almost pays for itself. Not long after
the Pontiac effort, the state of Michigan ordered all schools at
which at least 20 percent of students qualify for free meals to
offer breakfast.

Powell, who helped direct the Pontiac campaign, said it takes
only one or two parents to get started. She suggests building a
coalition of people from the PTA, the food service– workers'
union, churches, medical societies, and social-service agencies.

While forming your coalition, make an appointment with
the principal at your child's school. "The principal really has a
lot of authority to bring the program in," said Michele
Tingling-Clemmons, coordinator of FRAC's breakfast campaign. The principal may be able to tell you what obstacles are
blocking breakfast.

Early in the process, you also should meet with the district's
food service director. The director will have to implement the
breakfast program if the school board approves it. Again, you
may be able to learn what barriers you'll need to overcome. And
if you're lucky, you'll find a strong ally.

To sell breakfast, you need to show how it will help the
school. Telling school officials that breakfast can improve test
scores, make children better-behaved, and pay for itself may
pique their interest. "School breakfast is more than a nutrition
program, it's an education program," said Tingling-Clemmons.
"It prepares students to learn. That's the standpoint from which
you should approach it."

Ideally, your polite request will spur school officials immediately to start a breakfast program. If things are that easy, consider yourself blessed. "In most cases, it's a fight," said Henry
Shelton, who helps low-income parents in Rhode Island organize breakfast campaigns.

That's where the coalition you've been building comes in
handy. Ask the district superintendent to put you on the agenda

Where to Get Breakfast Help

I f you'd like to start a break-fast program, your strong-est ally will be the Food Research and Action Center in Washington, D.C. FRAC can provide all kinds of help in or-ganizing your campaign. It of-fers names of anti-hunger groups in your state that might help you, publications that ex-plain how to start a breakfast program and workshops.

Food Research and Action Center
1875 Connecticut Ave. NW
Suite 540
Washington, DC 20009
(202) 986-2200

for a school-board meeting. Then get as many people as possible to attend. Before the meeting, your coalition should decide exactly what it wants. Do you want a breakfast program districtwide? Do you want breakfast just in the neediest schools? Would you be willing to accept a pilot project in a few schools?

A few days before the meeting, call your local newspapers, radio stations, and TV stations to tell them you'll be speaking. Try to convince reporters to write an "advance" story about your campaign. Such a story has two advantages: It puts a little pressure on the board, and it alerts other people who may want to help you.

If the board questions the need for breakfast, you can gather statistics showing the need. Powell said you can find out from the school district how many children qualify for free and reduced-price lunches. You can make a case that families qualifying for lunch support often lack the money to feed their kids breakfast. You can get more statistical support from the U.S. Census Bureau's figures on poverty in your community (call 301-763-7662).

Teachers also can provide powerful testimony if they're willing to speak before the board. "We found that teachers usually know if they have hungry kids," Powell said.

If the board turns you down, step up your organizing. Expand your coalition, conduct a survey to measure community interest in a breakfast program, hold public meetings, and work with the media. And keep talking to school administrators and board members one-to-one.

Kathi Riley, a mother in Rhode Island, is part of Parents for Progress, a state-wide group that has been fighting for school breakfast programs. The group has obtained breakfast programs in Cranston and Pawtucket and is fighting for them in South Kingston. Riley says persistence is the key. "Take it one step at a time," she said. "Nobody's going to hand it to you. You're going to keep hitting brick walls, but just go around them and keep going and going and going."

Persuade the legislature to require schools statewide to offer breakfast. If you lose the breakfast battle locally, go to the legislature. That tactic has become increasingly successful.

"In the last several years, a number of states have passed mandates that require certain schools to offer the breakfast program," said Tingling-Clemmons. "Most mandates have required coalition efforts, and parents have been intimately involved in them." Most commonly, state laws require districts to offer breakfast if a certain percentage of students qualifies for free or reduced-price lunches.

Make sure the curriculum at your child's school includes a strong nutrition component. Whatever your child's grade level, the curriculum should include lessons on food and nutrition.

Parent-teacher conferences are a good time for you to ask what role nutrition plays in the curriculum. If there's little or no nutrition education, urge the teacher to do more. If the teacher lacks training in nutrition, you can suggest that he or she seek help from nutritionists at the county health department.

The school food service department may be able to help, too.

You should also check the nutrition units in any health textbooks your child uses. Many new textbooks are excellent, but some textbooks are woefully out of date.

You especially need to check any education materials produced by food companies. Teachers sometimes lack the time or knowledge needed to evaluate corporate materials, so you should check them yourself. For suggestions on what to look for, see the box on page 195 in Chapter 9. If you think the materials are misleading or deceptive, arrange a meeting with your child's teacher.

Other Steps to Take

Consider food when choosing a day-care center. Finding affordable day-care at all can be next to impossible. But if you have the luxury of choosing among centers, be sure to examine their meals.

Day-care facilities operate on extremely tight margins, so they try to save money wherever possible. You need to make sure they're not cutting corners on food. Even with limited funds, centers should be able to serve nutritious, tasty meals. There's no excuse for a center to serve hot dogs, french fries, and Kool-Aid every day.

Day-care centers with the strongest commitment to food often participate in the U.S. Department of Agriculture's Child Care Food Program. Under that program, both day-care centers and home-based facilities can get federal funding and commodities for meals. In 1993–94, the program provided a maximum of $2.735 per day in cash for each eligible child in a participating family day-care home. For large centers, there are some eligibility requirements based on income. But for day-care homes, every child qualifies regardless of income. In September 1991, more than 28,000 day-care centers and 177,000 day-care homes participated in the program.

You can learn much about how a center handles food by visiting at mealtime, said Mary Goodwin, former chief nutritionist for the Montgomery County Health Department in Maryland. She's been active in child-care food issues for more than 20 years.

Start by looking at what foods the center serves. "The meals should have a wide variety of whole grains, fruits and vegetables, low-fat dairy products, and lean fish or meat," Goodwin said. Some meals should feature vegetarian dishes with high-quality protein, she added.

Next, look at whether the portion sizes are appropriate for young children. Goodwin said some centers try to save money by serving measly portions.

Finally, you should see whether teachers are good role models during meals. The atmosphere in which teachers serve meals needs to be warm and nurturing, according to Goodwin, and teachers should eat with the children.

Be sure to ask lots of questions when you visit the center at mealtime. For a list of suggested questions, see the sidebar titled "Questions to Ask at a Day-Care Center" on the next page.

What if you're stuck with a day-care facility that serves junky food? Goodwin suggests organizing other parents. "Individually, you can be defeated," she said. Together, you may prevail.

Try to work with the day-care provider. Some simply lack the knowledge needed to provide high-quality meals. You can suggest that they seek help from a nutritionist at the local health department. You also can encourage them to participate in the federal Child Care Food Program (contact the Food and Nutrition Service, U.S. Department of Agriculture, 3101 Park Center Drive, Room 510, Alexandria, VA 22302).

Ultimately, you may only be able to get better food if you're willing to pay a little more. Goodwin acknowledges that most

Questions to Ask a Day-Care Center

When choosing a day-care center for your child, you should find out how it handles various food and nutrition issues. Here are questions that nutritionist Mary Goodwin suggests you should ask:

1. Does the center participate in and receive a subsidy from the federal Child Care Food Program?

2. Are meals prepared on-site?

3. Are children encouraged to help prepare the food?

4. Are children offered choices at meals?

5. Do the meals have a wide variety of whole grains, fruits and vegetables, low-fat dairy products, and lean meat, poultry, and fish?

6. Do the meals avoid foods high in fat, sugar, and sodium?

7. Do the meals avoid fried foods?

8. Does the staff eat with the children?

9. Has the staff received training in nutrition and feeding children?

10. Do parents get copies of menus?

11. Are parents welcome to visit during mealtimes?

12. At holidays, birthdays, and other celebrations, are healthy foods served?

13. If a child has a food problem, are the parents informed? How are such problems handled? Does the staff work with the parents to solve the problem?

14. Does the staff avoid using food as a reward or punishment?

15. Does the curriculum include lessons on food?

16. Are children exposed to ethnic foods and the accompanying cultures?

parents don't want to spend more on day care. To Goodwin, though, it's a choice of either paying extra for good food now or paying high doctors' bills later. Given that choice, spending more now becomes a real bargain.

Praise fast-food chains for offering healthier fare, and encourage them to do more. Many fast-food chains have started offering healthier foods in the last few years. What prompted the changes? Consumer pressure. What can cause more changes? More consumer pressure.

Write letters to the presidents of the fast-food chains you patronize, or talk to the restaurant managers. Tell them you appreciate the healthy improvements, and urge them to do more. Specifically, you should ask them to improve the nutritional quality of their packaged kids' meals. Ask them to include the lowest-fat sandwich possible (usually grilled chicken), to replace the fries with carrot sticks, and to trade the soft drink for 1-percent milk or orange juice.

Also, ask the chains to make nutrition information about their products easier to obtain. Suggest they print it on food wrappers, post it in their restaurants, or publish it in pamphlets provided free at each restaurant. Your town could also pass a law requiring them to post the calorie content of foods right next to the price on the menu board.

And finally, keep an eye on the chains' promotional campaigns. If you think their premiums are junky or their tactics are deceptive, write and tell them. We've listed addresses and telephone numbers for the major chains in the appendix titled "The Fast-Food Chains," page 283.

Urge your local television stations and the networks to run more pro-nutrition public-service announcements (PSAs) and programs. Local stations are sometimes responsive to their viewers, particularly if you organize a campaign that includes your school's PTA, the local chapters of the American Heart Association and the American Cancer Society, the state or local medical society, and others.

Ask the stations and networks to run pro-nutrition PSAs during programs aimed at kids, particularly on Saturday morning and weekday afternoons (if they don't have any PSAs on the shelf, ask that they work with you or a local college nutrition department to create one). Also, ask them to include segments on nutrition in programs aimed at kids or to create special programs about nutrition. You'd never realize it by watching them, but TV stations are licensed to operate in the public interest. Make them do so!

Monitor food commercials aimed at children. If you see a TV commercial that you think is unfair or deceptive, write letters to the Federal Trade Commission, your state's attorney general, and the Center for Science in the Public Interest. Also, urge your senators and member of Congress to support legislation that would strengthen the FTC's resolve to halt dishonest commercials. And finally, write or call the company whose product is advertised to express your displeasure.

After you write or call, urge your friends, PTA members, and others to do likewise. The more complaints the FTC, attorney general, or offending company gets, the more likely they are to pay attention.

More importantly, urge your legislators to support restrictions on junk-food ads. Alternatively, the government could pressure food advertisers and broadcasters to balance the junk-food ads with health messages.

Join local and national groups that are active in kids' food issues. While you possess some power as an individual parent, you can be much more powerful if you join with others. Simply put, there's strength in numbers.

At the local level, join the PTA at your child's school, an anti-hunger group, or the local chapter of the American Heart

An Agenda for Change

*T*hese are some of the measures that government and industry need to adopt to help your child, and every other child, eat a healthier diet.

• The Department of Agriculture should improve school breakfasts and lunches by setting limits on fat, sodium, and sugar. It should also provide more nutritious commodities to schools. As the government's chief agency for nutrition education, the USDA should provide advice for both kids and adults on choosing the most nutritious low-fat and vegetarian diets.

• The Department of Health and Human Services—in collaboration with city and state health departments—should mount major nutrition-education campaigns.

• The Surgeon General should publish periodic reports on children's nutrition.

• Congress should greatly increase funding for the School Lunch and Breakfast Programs to help schools offer more healthful meals. Congress also should pro- vide the funding necessary to make nutrition education a high priority in every school system.

• TV stations should increase greatly the number of health and nutrition programs and public-service announcements. The number of minutes devoted to nutrition messages should be at least as great as the number devoted to junk-food ads.

• Manufacturers should reformulate their products—especially those geared to kids—by improving the nutritional quality and omitting dyes and other questionable additives. Companies should also drop the phony kids "clubs," which are really just marketing devices.

• Supermarkets should be made "kid friendly" by eliminating candy displays at checkout counters, moving sugary cereals to upper shelves, carrying more healthy foods for kids, and offering nutrition education materials for children. They might copy one Maryland grocery store that has a "Fruit of the Week" club for children under 12; giving a child a free piece of fruit is a cheap way to encourage good eating habits and to have kids urging their parents to shop at that store. Supermarkets should also carry organic and other pesticide-free fresh and processed foods.

• Fast-food restaurants should offer prepackaged "kids' meals" that are especially nutritious. They might include low-fat burgers, carrot sticks, and orange juice.

• Schools should give nutrition the attention it deserves, both in the classroom and in the cafeteria. They should not allow the use of self-serving and misleading educational materials produced by the food industry.

• The federal government should sponsor new studies on the effects of diet on behavior.

• City and state governments should support organic farm-

ing, farmers' markets, and other means of increasing the supply of healthful, locally grown food.

• Government, industry, and private organizations should respond to the alarming increases in childhood obesity. Our society needs to mount a wide-ranging program involving bike paths, lower-calorie fast-food meals, an annual national "No-TV Week," more nutrition information and fewer junk-food ads on television, safer cities, and more physical education in schools. Such programs could be funded through small taxes on soft drinks, fast-food meals, and the $25 billion a year that the food-stamp program provides grocers.

• If you agree with any or all of these measures, get out your pen and paper and send a letter to your representative (Washington, DC 20515) and senators (Washington, DC 20510).

Association or the American Cancer Society. Try to interest those groups in kids' food issues. If one group isn't receptive, try another. And if you can't find a group that suits you, get some parents together and form your own.

There's also strength in numbers at the national level. Join the Center for Science in the Public Interest and Consumers Union. Both groups are very active on kids' food issues and can help you learn the issues yourself.

Your kids also can get involved. Nine-year-old Basil Schaheen of Derwood, Maryland, spoke at a nationally televised press conference that publicized the best—and worst—processed food for kids. Fourteen-year-old Camilla Jones of Oxford, Mississippi, compiled a computer database of all the ads that were broadcast in 20 hours of Saturday-morning television. She and 16-year-old Stephanie Marton of Arlington, Virginia, then participated in a press conference that criticized junk-food ads on children's television. Stephanie has been president and Basil vice-president of Kids Against Junk Food, a project of the Center for Science in the Public Interest. KAJF is an activist group that advocates a healthier food supply for kids. It has, for instance, written to President Clinton urging that he set a good example, rather than eating junky fast foods. KAJF also urged network TV executives to provide more nutrition public-service announcements and programs.

The projects we've listed above are just starting points for your own ideas. (For information on how to join the above-mentioned groups, see Appendix D, page 284.) Some efforts, like writing letters to fast-food companies, are simple things you can do by yourself. Others require joining with other people to pursue common goals. Even the largest projects, though, always start with one person. That person could be you.

Closing Thoughts

Clearly, your child's diet has a tremendous influence on his or her health. Food should be something that nourishes and helps your child grow stronger. Instead, all too often it promotes everything from tooth decay and obesity to heart disease and cancer. And the tragedy is that in too many ways children are actually encouraged to eat foods that are bad for their health.

Beyond health, food can be something that links children to the natural world, and meals can build stronger families. As food writer Nancy Harmon Jenkins put it, "Among life's greatest pleasures, after all, are those moments when we share with each other the sensuous delights of the table. These are the moments when strangers become friends and friends become lovers; when families become, in the fullest and richest sense, families; and when memories, strong, intense and persistent, are given birth."[1]

Getting your child to eat properly isn't a simple task. First, you need to make sure that *you* eat properly so the child can learn from your good example. That's more important than anything else. Then you have to encourage your child to develop tastes for healthier foods. And all the while, you have to battle all the bad influences—ranging from television commercials to premiums in cereal boxes to even the schools—that can lead your child astray.

Many parents are going one step further. Besides helping

their own children eat properly, they're also trying to improve the diets of all the kids in their child's school, their community, or the nation. They're doing everything from serving on PTA school-lunch committees to fighting for laws that will ensure that every baby has adequate nutrition.

The rewards of all that effort can be enormous. By teaching your own children about healthful food, you can be assured that—at a minimum—you gave them a healthy start in life. At best, you've helped protect them from a wide range of deadly diseases linked to food. And if you tackle projects outside your home, you get the satisfaction of knowing you've helped other children take the first steps down the path toward healthful eating as well.

We've tried in this book to explain why it's important for your kids to eat healthful diets. We hope that what you've learned helps you raise healthy kids who live long, happy lives.

Appendices and Endnotes

Appendices

Appendix A
USDA FOOD GUIDE PYRAMID

KEY

◼ Fat (naturally occurring and added)
▼ Sugars (added)

These symbols show that fat and added sugars come mostly from fats, oils, and sweets, but can be part of or added to foods from the other food groups as well.

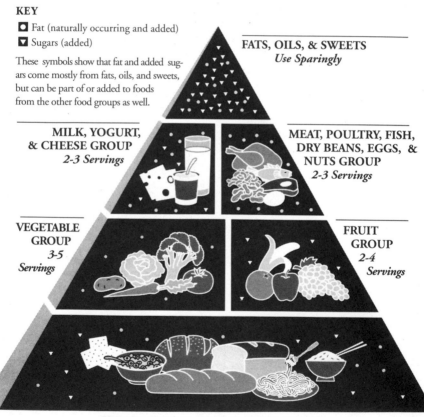

FATS, OILS, & SWEETS
Use Sparingly

MILK, YOGURT, & CHEESE GROUP
2-3 Servings

MEAT, POULTRY, FISH, DRY BEANS, EGGS, & NUTS GROUP
2-3 Servings

VEGETABLE GROUP
3-5 Servings

FRUIT GROUP
2-4 Servings

BREAD, CEREAL, RICE, & PASTA GROUP
6-11 Servings

SOURCE: U.S. Department of Agriculture/U.S. Department of Health and Human Services

What Counts as One Serving?

The following are what the USDA considers to be one serving, but the amount you eat may be more than one serving. For example, a dinner portion of spaghetti would count as two or three or even four servings of pasta.

Breads, Cereals, Rice, and Pasta
1 slice of bread
½ cup of cooked rice or pasta
½ cup of cooked cereal
1 ounce of ready-to-eat cereal

Vegetables
½ cup of chopped raw or cooked vegetables
1 cup of leafy raw vegetables

Fruits
1 piece of fruit or melon wedge
¾ cup of juice
½ cup of canned fruit
¼ cup of dried fruit

Meat, Poultry, Fish, Dry Beans, Eggs, and Nuts
2½ to 3 ounces of cooked lean meat, poultry, or fish
Count ½ cup of cooked beans, or 1 egg, or 2 tablespoons of peanut butter as 1 ounce of lean meat (about ⅓ serving)

Milk, Yogurt, and Cheese
1 cup of milk or yogurt
1½ to 2 ounces of cheese

Fats, Oils, and Sweets
Limit calories from these especially if you need to lose weight

Appendix B
CSPI'S HEALTHY EATING PYRAMID

Just as the U.S. Department of Agriculture has created a food guide pyramid, so has the Center for Science in the Public Interest. The difference is that CSPI's pyramid is four sided, presenting foods from every group divided into three categories—foods that one should eat anytime, sometimes, and seldom. (The fourth side provides nutrition information, here included below.) The pyramid also includes hard-to-categorize mixed foods, such as pizza, burritos, and canned soups. Owing to space limitations we could not reproduce the pyramid in its original form here, opting instead for a chart in a pyramid-like shape.

The best diets are rich in whole grains, beans, and fresh vegetables. They include only modest portions of low-fat animal foods like skim or 1 percent fat milk, yogurt, fish, and skinless chicken or turkey. (Vegetarians should replace meat with beans, peas, and lentils.) Here's how the pyramid can help you build a better diet:

Make *anytime* foods the backbone of your diet. With the exception of oily fish, they're low in fat and saturated fat, and have no serious flaws.

Limit *sometimes* foods to two or three a day or use small portions. Most contain moderate amounts of fat or saturated fat; a few are high in unsaturated fat. Others are high in sodium, cholesterol, or added sugar, or are made from white flour or white rice.

If you eat *seldom* foods, keep the portions small and/or limit them to two or three times a week. Most are high in fat or saturated fat. Others are moderate in fat, but have at least one other major flaw.

CSPI's pyramid originally was designed to be cut out and

Serving Sizes

The recommended number of daily servings of each food group are included in the Anytime pyramid. The following list provides typical serving sizes for older children and adults. Reduce the portion size for younger children.

Bread, Cereal, Rice, Pasta, and Baked Goods: 2 slices bread; ½ cup dense cereals (like granola); 1 cup other cooked cereal or pasta; ¾ cup cooked rice; 2 waffles; 3 pancakes; ⅒ cake; 1 oz. (2 to 3) cookies; ⅛ pie; ½ oz. (about 4) crackers; 1 oz. (about 14) chips.

Fish, Poultry, Meat, Nuts, and Eggs: 4 oz. cooked meat, poultry, or seafood; 1½ oz. shrimp; 3 oz. tuna; 2 oz. (two slices) luncheon meat; 1 hot dog; 1 egg; 2 Tb. peanut butter; ¼ cup nuts.

Vegetables and Beans: 1 cup lettuce; ½ cup cooked vegetables or beans.

Fruit: 1 medium fruit; ½ cup canned fruit; 1 cup juice.

Dairy Foods: 1 cup milk, yogurt, or ice cream; 1 oz. cheese; ½ cup cottage cheese.

Fats, Sweets, and Condiments: 1 Tb. margarine, butter, oil, catsup, mayonnaise, soy sauce, or jelly; 1 Tsp. mustard; 2 Tb. salad dressing.

Mixed Foods: 7 oz. (about 2 slices) pizza; 1 cup soup, cooked spaghetti, or chili.

assembled into a three-dimensional structure that could sit on a table top for ready reference. If you'd like a copy of this, CSPI offers full-color, 7-inch-high pyramids in sturdy paper for $4.00, or plastic for $15.00. Send a check to the Center for Science in the Public Interest, 1875 Connecticut Avenue, Suite 300, Washington, DC 20009-5728. Please include $2.00 for shipping and handling for each pyramid ordered.

CSPI's
Healthy Eating Pyramid I

ANYTIME

FATS, SWEETS, & CONDIMENTS
Ketchup; Olives;
Mustard; Mayonnaise, *fat-free*

DAIRY FOODS *(2 to 3 serving a day)*	**FISH, POULTRY, MEAT, NUTS, & EGGS** *(1 to 2 servings a day; trimmed; baked or roasted)*
Buttermilk; Cheese, *fat-free;* Cottage cheese, *fat-free or low-fat;* Milk, *skim or 1% fat;* Plain yogurt, *non-fat*	Seafood, *all;* Pork tenderloin; Tuna, *in water;* Chicken breast or drumstick, *no skin;* Egg white or substitute; Beef top or eye of round, *select;* Turkey, except wing, *no skin*
VEGETABLES & BEANS *(4 to 6 servings a day)*	**FRUITS** *(2 to 4 servings a day)*
Vegetables, *fresh, frozen, or canned;* Vegetable juice, *no-salt or light;* Beans (e.g., black, garbanzo, pink, pinto, great northern, kidney); Split peas; Lentils; Black-eyed peas	Fruit, *fresh, frozen, dried or canned with juice;* Fruit juice

BREAD, CEREALS, RICE, PASTA, & BAKED GOODS
(6 to 11 servings a day)
Bread, rolls, bagels; *whole-wheat or whole-grain;* Breakfast cereals, *cold, whole-grain, low-sugar* (e.g., bran flakes, Cheerios, Grape-Nuts, Life, Nutri-Grain, Shredded Wheat, Total, Wheaties); Breakfast cereals, *hot, whole-grain, low-sugar* (e.g., oatmeal, Wheatena); Bulgur; Corn tortillas; Crackers, *whole grain, low-fat* (e.g., crispbread, Triscuits); Pasta; Popcorn, *air-popped;* Rice, *brown;* Pretzels, *whole grain, unsalted;* Tortilla chips, *no-oil*

MIXED FOODS
Bean burrito; Cheeseless pizza; Grilled chicken sandwich;
Pork & beans; Garden salad with chicken chunks & light dressing; Canned soup, *low-sodium;* Spaghetti with tomato sauce; Vegetable pita sandwich; Stir-fried vegetables & rice with chicken or seafood; Turkey *(fresh-cooked)* sandwich

---

CSPI's
Healthy Eating Pyramid II

SOMETIMES

FATS, SWEETS, & CONDIMENTS
Jelly; Sugar; Oils;
Mayonnaise; Salad dressing;
Salt; Soy sauce; Margarine, *diet, tub*

DAIRY FOODS	FISH, POULTRY, MEAT, NUTS, & EGGS
Milk, *2% fat*; Sherbet; Ice milk; Ice cream, *non-fat*; Frozen yogurt, *all*; Cottage cheese, *4% fat*; Fruit yogurt, *non-fat or low-fat*; Cheese; Cream cheese; Sour cream, *light*	*(Trimmed; baked or roasted)* Turkey roll; Turkey, *w/skin*; tuna, *in oil*; Chicken nuggets; Nuts; Peanut butter; Pork loin (except blade); Beef round or sirloin steak; Chicken breast or drumstick, *w/skin*; Thigh, *no skin*
VEGETABLES & BEANS	**FRUITS**
Avocado; Cole slaw; French fries; Guacamole; Hash browns; Potato chips; Corn chips; Potato salad; V8 juice; Tomato juice, *canned*; Soybeans; Tofu	Cranberry sauce, *canned* ; Fruit, *canned in syrup*; Fruit "drinks," "blends," "cocktails," or "beverages"

BREADS, CEREAL, RICE, PASTA, & BAKED GOODS
Angelfood cake; Fig bars; Pancakes; Waffles; Oatmeal raisin cookies; Gingersnaps; Molasses cookies; Pretzels; Rice, *white;* Packaged rice mixes; Tortilla chips, *light*; Bread, rolls, bagels, *multi-grain, oatmeal, rye, pumpernickel, white;* Biscuits; Croissants; Cakes; Cookies; Granola bars, *fat-free*; Breakfast cereals, *refined* (e.g., corn flakes, Rice Krispies); Crackers, *refined* (e.g., saltines, oyster); Crackers, *not low-fat* (e.g., cheese, Ritz); Breakfast cereals, *heavily sweetened* (e.g., Cap'n Crunch, Frosted Flakes)

MIXED FOODS
Baked potato w/cheese; Beef or chicken burrito; Canned or dried soup; Cheese pizza; Chef salad w/ light dressing; Chicken taco; Hummus w/pita; Lasagna w/meat; McLean Deluxe; Macaroni & cheese; Peanut butter & jelly sandwich; Roast beef sandwich; Spaghetti w/meatballs; Tuna or chicken salad sandwich

CSPI's
Healthy Eating Pyramid III

SELDOM

**FATS, SWEETS, &
CONDIMENTS**
Chocolate; Butter;
Margarine, *stick*

DAIRY FOODS	**FISH, POULTRY, MEAT, NUTS, & EGGS** *(Trimmed; baked or roasted)*
Milk, *whole*; Cheesecake; Yogurt, *whole-milk*; Ice cream, *regular or gourmet*; Cheese (e.g., Cheddar, Swiss, American)	Eggs; Ribs; Ham; Bologna; Red meat, *untrimmed;* Chicken thigh or wing, *with skin*; Hot dog, *turkey or meat*; Beef steaks or roasts, most types, *choice*; Ground beef, *regular*
VEGETABLES & BEANS	**FRUITS**
Onion rings; Potatoes *au gratin*; Vegetables *with hollandaise sauce*	Coconut

BREADS, CEREAL, RICE, PASTA, & BAKED GOODS
Apple pie, *fried*; Bread stuffing from mix; Cake (*except fat-free*) with frosting;
Chocolate chip cookies; Chocolate sandwich cookies; Cream pie; Danishes;
Doughnuts; Granola bars (*except fat-free*); Lemon meringue pie; Peanut butter
cookies; Pecan pie; Shortbread cookies

MIXED FOODS
Bologna sandwich; Chef salad with regular dressing; Double hamburger or cheeseburger; Chili; French toast w/ syrup; Grilled cheese sandwich; Ham & cheese sandwich; Hot dog on bun; Nachos w/ cheese; Pizza, *pepperoni or sausage;* Quarter-pound
hamburger or Cheeseburger; Beef taco; Taco salad

Appendix C
THE FAST-FOOD CHAINS

Arby's
6917 Collins Avenue
Miami Beach, FL 33141
(800) 223-8473

Burger King Corporation
P.O. Box 520783
General Mail Facility
Miami, FL 33152-0783
(800) 937-1800

Carl Karcher Enterprises
P.O. Box 4349
Anaheim, CA 92803
(714) 774-5796

Dairy Queen/Brazier
5701 Green Valley Drive
P.O. Box 35286
Minneapolis, MN 55435
(612) 830-0200

Domino's Pizza Inc.
30 Frank Lloyd Wright Drive
P.O. Box 997
Ann Arbor, MI 48106-0997
(313) 930-3030

Hardee's Food Systems Inc.
1233 North Church Street
Rocky Mount, NC 27801
(800) 346-2243

Jack in the Box
Foodmaker Inc.
P.O. Box 783
San Diego, CA 92112-4126
(619) 571-2121

KFC (Kentucky Fried Chicken)
P.O. Box 32070
Louisville, KY 40232-2070
(502) 456-8300

Long John Silver's
Jerrico Inc.
P.O. Box 11988
Lexington, KY 40579
(800) 735-5555

McDonald's
McDonald's Plaza
Oak Brook, IL 60521
(708) 575-FOOD

Pizza Hut
P.O. Box 428
Wichita, KS 67201
(316) 681-9000

Popeye's/Church's Fried Chicken
1333 S. Clearview Parkway
Jefferson, LA 70121
(504) 733-4300

Roy Rogers Restaurants
c/o Hardee's Food Systems Inc.
1233 North Church Street
Rocky Mount, NC 27801
(800) 346-2243

Subway
325 Bic Drive
Milford, CT 06460
(800) 888-4848

Taco Bell Corporation
17901 Von Karman
Irvine, CA 92714
(800) 225-8226; (714) 863-4500

Wendy's International Inc.
P.O. Box 256
Dublin, OH 43017
(614) 764-3100

Appendix D
GROUPS TO JOIN, PUBLICATIONS TO GET

Center for Science in the Public Interest
1875 Connecticut Avenue NW,
Suite 300
Washington, DC 20009-5728
Annual membership: $24

For more than two decades, CSPI has worked to improve the nation's diet and health. It has undertaken numerous activities specifically aimed at children, including pressuring fast-food restaurants and schools to improve their foods.

Membership includes a subscription to *Nutrition Action Healthletter,* a lively newsletter that provides current information on nutrition and food safety.

Kids Against Junk Food
Center for Science in the Public Interest
1875 Connecticut Avenue NW,
Suite 300
Washington, DC 20009-5728

Kids Against Junk Food is a group of elementary and high school kids who eat healthy diets and want to help others do the same. KAJFers have spoken at press conferences, written complaints to junk-food producers, and appeared on national TV shows.

Members of KAJF care about —and *do* something about—the nutritional quality of school meals, TV commercials for junk foods, environmental effects of overpackaged foods, and hunger.

Kids, teachers, or parents who are interested in starting a local chapter of KAJF should send $1 to the above address for a CHOW! (Children for Healthy Food and a Healthy World) Club Hands-on Handbook. The handbook offers a myriad of fun, nutrition-related activties.

Consumer Reports
Subscription Department
P.O. Box 51166
Boulder, CO 80321-1166

Zillions
Subscription Department
P.O. Box 51777
Boulder, CO 80321-1777

The Consumers Union publishes *Consumer Reports* magazine and *Zillions: Consumer Reports for Kids. Zillions,* which just like *Consumer Reports* provides unbiased information about products, is aimed at kids ages 8 to 14. Both publications have frequent articles about food and nutrition. One year of *Consumer Reports* costs $22, while one year of *Zillions* costs $16.

Mothers & Others for a Livable Planet
40 W. 20th Street
New York, NY 10011
Annual membership: $15

Mothers & Others is an offshoot of the Natural Resources Defense Coucil, one of the nation's premier environmental groups. Mothers & Others focuses on the risks of pesticides, lead, and other environmental problems that threaten children's health. Members receive a quarterly newsletter.

Endnotes

Introduction: Feeding Our Kids Right—What Could Be More Important?

1. Frances R. Davidson et al., "Towards Accurate Assessment of Children's Food Consumption," *Ecology of Food and Nutrition* 18 (1986), 309.

2. Nationwide Food Consumption Survey, Human Nutrition Information Service, U.S. Department of Agriculture, 1985.

3. G. C. Frank et al., "Dietary Studies and the Relationship of Diet to Cardiovascular Disease Risk Factor Variables in 10-Year-Old Children—The Bogalusa Heart Study," *The American Journal of Clinical Nutrition* (February 1978), 333.

4. James Blaylock and Noel Blisard, "Slow Growth in Food Spending Expected," *Food Review,* U.S. Department of Agriculture, Economic Research Service, Vol. 16, No. 2 May–August, 1993, 2.

5. "Food Away From Home and the Quality of the Diet," *Food Review,* U.S. Department of Agriculture, Economic Research Service (Winter 1984), 14.

6. "What Is America Eating?" (Proceedings of a Symposium, Food and Nutrition Board, National Research Council, National Academy Press, 1986), 112.

7. Gladys Block and Bill Patterson, "Food Choices and the Cancer Guidelines," *American Journal of Public Health* 78 (1988), 282.

8. The Kellogg Children's Nutrition Survey: Executive Summary, June 1989, table 3.

9. Ibid., table 14.

10. Ibid., table 1.

11. Ibid., table 9.

12. American School Health Association et al., The National Adolescent Student Health Survey, (Oakland, CA: Third Party Publishing, 1989), 111.

13. Kellogg Nutrition Survey, table 11.

Chapter 1: Fat and Cholesterol

1. *The Surgeon General's Report on Nutrition and Health,* Public Health Service, U.S. Department of Health and Human Services (1988), 2.

2. William Enos et al., "Coronary Disease Among United States Soldiers Killed in Action in Korea: Preliminary Report," *JAMA,* 152 (1953), 1090.

3. Alden Manchester, "Food Spending Grows Slowly," *Food Review* 16 No. 3, (1993) table 1, 23.

4. *Report of the Expert Panel on Blood Cholesterol Levels in Children and Adolescents,* National Cholesterol Education Program, National Heart, Lung, and Blood Institute, U.S. Department of Health and Human Services (March 27, 1991), 10.

5. William P. Newman III et al., "Relation of Serum Lipoprotein Levels and Systolic Blood Pressure to Early Atherosclerosis: The Bogalusa Heart Study," *The New England Journal of Medicine* 314 (1986), 138.

6. "Relationship of Atherosclerosis in Young Men to Serum Lipoprotein Cholesterol Concentrations and Smoking: A Preliminary Report from the Pathobiological Determinants of Atherosclerosis in Youth (PDAY) Research Group," *JAMA,* 264, (1990), 3018.

7. "Daily Dietary Fat and Total Food-Energy Intakes–Third National Health and Nutrition Survey, Phase 1" *Morbidity & Mortality Weekly Report* 43 (1994), 110-25.

8. While 30 percent fat may be a reasonable target for children, many experts are urging the general public to limit fat to 25 percent, 20 percent, or even less.

9. Frances E. Thompson and Barbara Dennison, "Dietary Sources of Fat and Cholesterol in Children Aged 2 Through 5 Years," *American Journal of Public Health* 84 (May 1994), 799.

10. *"Daily Dietary Fat and Total Food-Energy Intakes,"* 110–25.

11. Walter C. Willett and Albert Ascherio, *"Trans* Fatty Acids: Are the Effects Only Marginal?" *American Journal of Public Health* 84 (1994), 722.

12. George A. Bray, *Recent Advances in Obesity Research* 2 (1978), 221.

13. Theresa A. Nicklas et al., "Nutrient Adequacy of Low Fat Intakes for Children: The Bogalusa Heart Study," *Pediatrics* 89 (1992), 221–228.

14. Gilbert Martinez and Alan Ryan, "What Are Children in the United States Eating?" in *Prevention of Adult Atherosclerosis During Childhood,* Report of the 95th Ross Conference on Pediatric Research, 1988, 55.

15. John Morrison et al., "Interrelationships between Nutrient Intake and Plasma Lipids and Lipoproteins in Schoolchildren Aged 6 to 19: The Princeton School District Study," *Pediatrics,* 65 (1980), 730.

16. "What Are Children in the United States Eating?" 59.

17. *Diet, Nutrition & Cancer Prevention: A Guide to Food Choices,* National Cancer Institute, NIH Publication No. 87-2878 (May 1987), 39.

18. *The Surgeon General's Report on Nutrition and Health,* 194.

19. *Diet and Health: Implications for Reducing Chronic Disease Risk,* National Research Council, Committee on Diet and Health (1989), 7–113.

20. American Cancer Society, *Cancer Facts & Figures—1993* (1993), 7.

21. John H. Weisburger, "Causes, Relevant Mechanisms, and Prevention of Large Bowel Cancer," *Seminars on Oncology* 18 (1991), 316.

22. Walter C. Willett et al., "Relationship of Meat, Fat, and Fiber Intake in the Risk of Colon Cancer in a Prospective Study Among Women," *New England Journal of Medicine,* 323 (1990), 1664.

23. Edward Giovannucci et al., "Relationship of Diet to Risk of Colorectal Adenoma in Men," *Journal of the National Cancer Institute* 84 (1992), 91.

24. Edward Giovannucci, "A Prospective Study of Dietary Fat and Risk of Prostate Cancer," *Journal of the National Cancer Institute* 85 (1993), 1571.

25. *Cancer Facts & Figures—1993,* 7.

26. *Reducing Chronic Disease Risk,* 7–78.

Chapter 2: Sugar and Salt

1. *Evaluation of Health Aspects of Sugars Contained in Carbohydrate Sweeteners,* Report of Sugars Task Force, U.S. Food and Drug Administration (1986), S28.

2. Letter to Bruce Maxwell from Ann Bouchoux, The Sugar Association Inc., 7 September 1990.

3. Report of Sugars Task Force, S26, S31.

4. Patricia M. Guenther, "Beverages in the Diets of American Teenagers," *Journal of the American Dietetic Association* 86 (1986), 493.

5. S. Kashket et al., "Lack of Correlation between Food Retention on the Human Dentition and Consumer Perception of Food Stickiness," *Journal of Dental Research* 70 (1991), 1314.

6. Press release from National Institutes of Health, 21 June 1988.

7. Estner H. Wender and M. V. Solanto, "Effects of Sugar on Aggressive and Inattentive Behavior in Children with Attention Deficit Disorder with Hyperactivity and Normal Children," *Pediatrics* 88 (1991), 960.

8. J. A. Goldman et al., "Behavioral Effects of Sucrose on Preschool Children," *Journal of Abnormal Child Psychology* 14 (1986), 565–77.

9. J. L. Rapoport, "Effects of Dietary Substances in Children," *Journal of Psychiatric Research* 17 (1982/83), 187–191; M.J.P. Kreusi and J. L. Rapoport, "Diet and Human Behavior: How Much Do They Affect Each Other?" *Annual Review of Nutrition* 6 (1986), 113–30.

10. Mark L. Wohlraich et al., "Effects of Diets High in Sucrose or Aspartame on the Behavior and Cognitive Performance of Children," *New England Journal of Medicine* 330 (1994), 301.

11. *1993 Heart and Stroke Facts Statistics,* American Heart Association.

12. *Recommended Dietary Allowances,* 10th ed., Food and Nutrition Board, National Academy of Sciences (1989), 253.

13. Ernst Wynder, ed., *Cholesterol: A Pediatric Perspective,* Practice of Surgery Ltd. (1989), 12.

14. Calculations based on sodium intake data from the Bogalusa Heart Study and requirements from the *Recommended Dietary Allowances.*

15. *Recommended Dietary Allowances,* 251.

16. Ailsa Goulding, "Osteoporosis: Why Consuming Less Sodium Chloride Helps to Conserve Bone," *New Zealand Medical Journal* 103 (1990), 120 ; B. E. Christopher et al., "The Nature and Significance of the Relationship between Urinary Sodium and Urinary Calcium in Women," *Journal of Nutrition* 123 (1993), 1615.

17. Pelayo Correa, "Diet Modification and Gastric Cancer Prevention," *Journal of the National Cancer Institute Monograph* 12 (1992), 75.

18. *Diet and Health: Implications for Reducing Chronic Disease Risk,* National Research Council, Committee on Diet and Health (1989), 15–18.

Chapter 3: The Obesity Epidemic

1. S. L. Gortmaker et al., "Increasing Pediatric Obesity in the United States," *American Journal of Diseases of Children,* 141 (1987), 535–40.

2. Charles Shear et al., "Secular Trends of Obesity in Early Life: The Bogalusa Heart Study," *American Journal of Public Health* 78 (1988), 77.

3. Chandra M. Tiwary et al., "Prevalence of Obesity Among Children of Military Dependents at Two Major Medical Centers," *American Journal of Public Health* 82 (1992), 354.

4. *1990 Report on Television,* Nielsen Media Research (1990) 8.

5. William Dietz et al., "Do We Fatten Our Children at the Television Set? Obesity and Television Viewing in Children and Adolescents," *Pediatrics* 75 (1985), 807.

6. R. C. Klesges et al., "Effects of Television on Metabolic Rate: Potential Implications for Childhood Obesity," *Pediatrics* 91 (1993), 281.

7. *The Surgeon General's Report on Nutrition and Health,* U.S. Department of Health and Human Services, DHHS Publication No. 88-50210 (1988), 287.

8. A. V. Must et al., "Long-term Morbidity and Morbidity of Overweight Adolescents," *New England Journal of Medicine* 327 (1992), 1350.

9. Quoted in "The Relationship between Nutrition & Learning," National Education Association, Washington (1989), 23.

10. Leonard Epstein et al., "Childhood Obesity," *Pediatric Clinics of North America* 32, (1985), 364.

11. *Diet and Health: Implications for Reducing Chronic Disease Risk,* National Research Council, Committee on Diet and Health (1989), 21–35.

12. Ibid.

13. A. J. Stunkard et al., "The Body-Mass Index of Twins Who Have Been Reared Apart," *New England Journal of Medicine* 322 (1990), 1483–7.

14. *Reducing Chronic Disease Risk,* 5–32.

15. M.K. Serdula, "Weight Control Practices of U.S. Adolescents and Adults," *Annals of Internal Medicine* 119 (1993), 667.

16. *The Surgeon General's Report,* 522.

17. Ibid., 510.

18. C. Johnson et al., "Incidence and Correlates of Bulimic Behavior in a Female High School Population," *Journal of Youth and Adolescence* 13 (1984), 15.

19. Paula Howat and Arnold Saxton, "The Incidence of Bulimic Behavior in a Secondary and University School Population," *Journal of Youth and Adolescence* 17, No. 3 (1988), 221.

Chapter 4: Bacteria, Additives, and Pesticides

1. Frank E. Young, "Food Safety and FDA's Action Plan Phase II," *Food Technology* 41 (November 1987), 116.

2. For a more thorough discussion of food safety, see: Michael F. Jacobson, Lisa Y. Lefferts, and Anne Witte Garland, *Safe Food: Eating Wisely in a Risky World,* (Living Planet Press (Venice, California, 1991).

3. *Diet and Health: Implications for Reducing Chronic Disease Risk,* National Research Council, Committee on Diet and Health (1989), 17–43.

4. *Reducing Chronic Disease Risk,* 1–15.

5. *Safe Food,* 155.

6. A. J. Zametkin et al., "Cerebral Glucose Metabolism in Adults with Hyperactivity of Childhood Onset," *New England Journal of Medicine* 323 (1990), 1361–6.

7. *Reducing Chronic Disease Risk,* 17–22.

8. James M. Swanson and Marcel Kinsbourne, "Food Dyes Impair Performance of Hyperactive Children on a Laboratory Learning Test," *Science* 207 (1980), 1485–7.

9. Ibid., 1487.

10. Bernard Weiss, "Food Additive Safety Evaluation," *Advances in Child Psychology* 7 (1984), 221–251.

11. Bonnie J. Kaplan et al., "Dietary Replacement in Preschool-aged Hyperactive Boys," *Pediatrics* 83 (1989), 7–17.

12. Marvin Boris and Francine S. Mandel, "Foods and Additives are Common Causes of the Attention Deficit Hyperactive Disorder in Children," *Annals of Allergy* 72 (1994), 462–8.

13. Bernard Weiss, "Food Additives as a Source of Behavioral Disturbances in Children," *NeuroToxicology* 7 (1986), 197–208.

14. J. L. Rapoport, "Effects of Dietary Substances on Children," *Journal of Psychiatric Research* 17 (1982/83), 187–91.

15. Judith L. Rapoport et al., "Behavioral and Cognitive Effects of Caffeine in Boys and Adult Males," *Journal of Nervous and Mental Disease* 169 (1981), 726; Judith L. Rapoport et al., "Behavioral Effects of Caffeine in Children," *Archives of General Psychiatry* 41 (1984), 1073.

16. *Regulating Pesticides in Food: The Delaney Paradox,* Board on Agriculture, National Research Council (Washington, D.C.: National Academy Press, 1987), 56.

17. L. Lefferts, *Nutrition Action Healthletter* Vol. 16, No. 3 (1989), 5; quoting Donald Reed of the FDA.

18. David Pimentel, ed., *CRC Handbook of Pest Management in Agriculture,* 2nd ed., vol. 1 (CRC Press Inc., 1991), 679.

19. Testimony of Fred Shank, director of the Center for Food Safety and Applied Nutrition, U.S. Department of Agriculture, at *Safety of Pesticides in Food: Hearing before the Subcommittee on Health and the Environment of the Committee on Energy and Commerce, House of Representatives* (June 19, 1991), Serial No. 102-35, 92.

20. Ibid.

21. *The Delaney Paradox,* 49.

22. *Unfinished Business: A Comparative Assessment of Environmental Problems,* Overview Report, U.S. Environmental Protection Agency, Office of Policy Analysis (February 1987), 84.

23. *The Delaney Paradox,* 65.

24. *Safety of Pesticides in Food: Hearing before the Subcommittee on Health and the Environment of the Committee on Energy and Commerce, House of Representatives* (June 19, 1991), Serial No. 102-35, 348.

25. *Intolerable Risk: Pesticides in our Children's Food,* Natural Resources Defense Council (February 27, 1989), 4.

26. *For Our Kids' Sake,* Natural Resources Defense Council, New York (1989), 17.

27. *Safety of Pesticides in Food,* 205, 208.

28. Ibid., 116.

29. *Intolerable Risk,* 6.

30. *The Delaney Paradox,* 61.

31. Ibid., 41.

32. *Pesticides in the Diets of Infants and Children,* National Research Council, 1993, 7–8.

33. "Food Safety: Difficulties in Assessing Pesticides Risks and Benefits," statement of John Harman before the Subcommittee on Department Operations, Research, and Foreign Agriculture, Committee on Agriculture, House of Representatives, GAO/T-RCED-92-33 (February 26, 1992), 5.

34. Statement by Rep. Henry Waxman, *Safety of Pesticides in Food: Hearing before the Subcommittee on Health and the Environment of the Committee on Energy and Commerce, House of Representatives* (June 19, 1991), Serial No. 102-35, 103.

35. "Pesticides in Children's Diets: What Are the Risks?" statement by Richard Jackson, American Academy of Pediatrics, Plenary Session, New Orleans, Louisiana (October 18, 1991).

36. *Safety of Pesticides in Food,* 207.

37. *CRC Handbook of Pest Management in Agriculture,* 679.

38. Ibid., 707.

39. Ibid., 681–2.

40. "Pesticides in Children's Diets."

Chapter 5: Eat Your Veggies . . . and Other Good Foods

1. Ellen Haas, Testimony, September 13, 1993, House Subcommittee on Human Resources and Intergovernmental Relations.

2. "Fruits and Vegetables—Not!" *U.S. News and World Report,* (May 9, 1994), 18.

3. Edward Giovannucci et al., "Relationship of Diet to Risk of Colorectal Adenoma in Men," *Journal of the National Cancer Institute* 84 (1992), 34.

4. Victor Fulgoni and Maureen Mackey, "Total Dietary Fiber in Children's Diets," (undated paper), 4.

5. *Diet, Nutrition & Cancer Prevention: A Guide to Food Choices,* National Cancer Institute, NIH Publication No. 87-2878 (May 1987), 4.

6. *Diet, Nutrition & Cancer Prevention: The Good News,* National Cancer Institute, NIH Publication No. 87-2878 (December 1986).

7. David Schardt, "Phytochemicals: Plants Against Cancer," *Nutrition Action Healthletter* Vol. 21, No. 3, (1994) 1.

Chapter 6: How Food Companies Seduce Kids

1. Tim Kelly, "At Washington State, Fast Food Now Offered as Course of Study: Professor's Chair Endowed by Taco Bell," *The Washington Post,* January 12, 1989, D13.

2. Valerie Reitman, "Marketing: Those Little Kids Have Big Pockets," *The Wall Street Journal,* August 26, 1992, B1.

3. Patricia Sellers, "The ABC's of Marketing to Kids," *Fortune,* May 8, 1989, 114.

4. Ibid.

5. Carol Hall, "Tween Power: Youth's Middle Tier Comes of Age," *Marketing & Media Decisions*, October 1987, 56; and "The ABC's of Marketing to Kids," 114.

6. "The ABC's of Marketing to Kids," 114.

7. "Tween Power: Youth's Middle Tier Comes of Age," 56.

8. David J. Morrow, "Picking Junior's Pocket," *The Marketer* (May 1990), 20.

9. "Tween Power: Youth's Middle Tier Comes of Age," 56.

10. *FTC Staff Report on Television Advertising to Children,* Federal Trade Commission (February 1978), 1.

11. Interview with Michael Evans.

12. Leslie Ellis, "Kids and Buying Decisions," The Louisville *Courier-Journal*, February 5, 1990, 1C.

13. Cited in "Kids and Buying Decisions."

14. *Burger King Corporation Fast Facts for the 90's,* Burger King Corporation, undated.

15. Paul Nolan, "Turtles Spearhead Whopper of a Promotion for Burger," *Promotion Marketing* (June 1990), 1.

16. Kate Fitzgerald and Julie Liesse, "Jetsons Fly Into Hot Licensing Year," *Advertising Age,* July 16, 1990, 43.

17. Christine Donahue, "Ralston Cereal Gets a Lift From *Ghostbusters II*," *Adweek's Marketing Week,* July 3, 1989, 28.

18. James S. Hirsch, "Fast-Food Vendors Get Serious With Kids," *The Wall Street Journal,* January 20, 1990, B1.

19. Rajan Chaudhry, "Lights, Cameras, Fast Food: Top Chains Bank on Movie Tie-ins," *Nation's Restaurant News,* June 19, 1989, 1.

20. Cara Appelbaum, "If Kiddie Ads Need Restraint, What About the Turtles?" *Adweek's Marketing Week,* October 8, 1990, 5.

21. Ibid.

22. *The Market for Breakfast Foods,* Business Trends Analysts Inc. (1989), 339-40.

23. "Move Over, Cap'n Crunch: Pac-Man and His Pals Are Taking Over," *Business Week,* July 18, 1983, 174.

24. Joseph Pereira, "Kids' Advertisers Play Hide-and-Seek, Concealing Commercials in Every Cranny," *The Wall Street Journal,* April 30, 1990, B1, B6.

25. *Selling America's Kids: Commercial Pressures on Kids of the 90's,* Consumers Union (1990), 5.

26. Randall Rothenberg, "Is It a Film? Is It an Ad? Harder to Tell," *The New York Times,* 23 March 1990, D23.

27. J. D. Reed, "Plugging Away in Hollywood," *Time,* January 2, 1989, 103.

28. *Selling America's Kids*, 18, and *Brand-Name References in the Top-Grossing Movies of 1990*, Center for the Study of Commercialism (May 30, 1991).

29. *In the Matter of Unfair and Deceptive Acts and Practices in the Placement of Product Advertisements in Motion Pictures*, filed with the Federal Trade Commission by the Center for the Study of Commercialism (May 30, 1991), exhibit 1.

30. *Selling America's Kids*, 18, and *Brand-Name References in the Top-Grossing Movies of 1990*.

31. *In the Matter of Unfair and Deceptive Acts and Practices in the Placement of Product Advertisements in Motion Pictures*, exhibit 4.

32. Ibid., exhibit 3.

33. Ibid, 12.

34. Sharon Warren Walsh, "Toy Promotions Are Serious Business for Fast-Food Chains," *The Washington Post*, December 11, 1987, D8.

35. Charles Atkin, "Effects of Television Advertising on Children," in *Children and the Faces of Television: Teaching, Violence, Selling*, ed. Edward Palmer and Aimee Door (San Diego: Academic Press, 1981), 287.

36. Charles Atkin, *Effects of Television Advertising on Children: Parent Child Communication in Supermarket Breakfast Selection*, Report 7 (Michigan State University, 1975).

37. "Fast-Food Vendors Get Serious With Kids."

38. Sherry Beck Paprocki, "The Fast-Food Wooing of Your Children," *Columbus Monthly* (April 1989), 139.

39. George Lazarus, "Sears Has Whopper in McKids," *Adweek*, May 4, 1987, 28.

Chapter 7: Television, the Sneaky Salesmachine

1. *FTC Staff Report on Television Advertising to Children*, Federal Trade Commission (February 1978), 13.

2. *1990 Report on Television*, A. C. Nielsen Company (1990), 8.

3. *Children and Advertising Fact Sheet*, Consumers Union, undated (1990).

4. Testimony of Bruce Watkins, *Hearings before the Subcommittee on Telecommunications and Finance of the Committee on Energy and Commerce, House of Representatives, on H.R. 3288, H.R. 3966, and H.R. 4125*, 100th Congress, Serial No. 100-93, September 15, 1987, and March 17, 1988, 326.

5. Ibid., 325.

6. *Research on the Effects of Television Advertising on Children*, National Science Foundation (1977), 99.

7. *Television Advertising to Children: Message Content in 1990*, Children's Advertising Review Unit, Council of Better Business Bureaus (January 1991), 24.

8. Shawn Tully, "What CEO's Really Make," *Fortune,* June 15, 1992, 95.

9. Thomas J. Stare, Lisa C. Cohn, Robert A. MacIntosh, and Richard J. Deckelbaum, "Children's Television Commercials and Recommendations for Dietary Fat Intake," *Abstracts from the 66th Scientific Sessions* (Abstract #62), American Heart Association, 8 November 1993.

10. Gary Levin, "Cost of TV Spot Pegged at $145,000," *Advertising Age,* 6 March 1989, 68, quoting figures from the American Association of Advertising Agencies.

11. "Top 25 Network TV Advertisers" and "Top 25 Spot TV Advertisers," *Advertising Age,* September 29, 1993, 44, 46.

12. Robert M. Liebert and Joyce Sprafkin, *The Early Window: Effects of Television on Children and Youth* (New York: Pergamon Press, 1988), 168.

13. C. Atkin and W. Gibson, "Children's Nutrition Learning from Television Advertising" (unpublished manuscript, Michigan State University, 1978).

14. WTTG, Channel 5, Washington, D.C. (April 26, 1991).

15. Dale Kunkel, "Children and Host-Selling Television Commercials," *Communication Research* (February 1988), 72.

16. *Television Advertising to Children: Message Content in 1990,* 20–2.

17. Charles Atkin, "Effects of Television Advertising on Children," in *Children and the Faces of Television: Teaching, Violence, Selling,* ed. Edward Palmer and Aimee Door (San Diego: Academic Press, 1981), 288.

18. Ibid., 295–6.

19. Ibid.

20. Nancy Signorielli, "Health and the Media: Images and Impact," paper commissioned for Mass Communications and Health: Complexities and Conflicts (September 17–19, 1988), 22.

21. *Television Advertising to Children: Message Content in 1990,* 24.

22. Michael Geis, *The Language of Television Advertising* (San Diego: Academic Press, 1982), 209.

23. *Self-Regulatory Guidelines for Children's Advertising,* Children's Advertising Review Unit, Council of Better Business Bureaus, 4th edition (1991), 4.

24. "Children's Nutrition Learning from Television Advertising."

25. *Television Advertising to Children: Message Content in 1990,* 45.

26. *Self-Regulatory Guidelines for Children's Advertising,* 7.

27. *Television Advertising to Children: Message Content in 1990,* 45, 52.

28. Charles Atkin, *Effects of Television Advertising on Children: Survey of Children's and Mothers' Responses to Television Commercials,* Technical Report (Michigan State University, 1975).

29. James U. McNeal, *Children as Consumers: Insights and Implications* (New York: Lexington Books, 1987), 124–5.

30. *Television Advertising to Children: Message Content in 1990,* 27.

31. Debra Scammon and Carole Christopher, "Nutrition Education with Children Via Television: A Review," *Journal of Advertising,* Vol. 10 (2) (1981), 26–36.

32. *Edible TV: Your Child and Food Commercials,* prepared by the Council on Children, Media and Merchandising for the Senate Committee on Nutrition and Human Needs, 95th Congress, 1st session (September 1977), 69–70.

33. *FTC Staff Report on Television Advertising to Children,* 94.

34. Joann Paley Galset and Mary Alice White, "The Unhealthy Persuader: The Reinforcing Value of Television and Children's Purchase-Influencing Attempts at the Supermarket," *Child Development* (1976), Vol. 47, 1089–96.

35. *FTC Staff Report on Television Advertising to Children,* 95–6.

36. Charles Atkin, *Effects of Television Advertising on Children: Survey of Preadolescents' Responses to Television Commercials,* Technical Report (Michigan State University, 1975).

37. *Children's Television Act of 1989, Report Together With Dissenting Views,* Report 101-385, 101st Congress, House of Representatives (November 21, 1989), 5.

38. Action for Children's Television v. FCC, 821 F.2nd 741 at 747, quoted in *Children's Television Act of 1989,* Report 101-385, 4.

39. Action for Children's Television v. FCC, 821 F.2nd 741, 744, quoted in *Children's Television Act of 1989,* Report 101–385, 5; and *Children's Television Act of 1989,* Report 101-227, Committee on Commerce, Science, and Transportation, 101st Congress, 5.

40. *FTC Staff Report on Television Advertising to Children,* 27.

41. Ibid., 29.

42. Ibid., 10, 24.

43. *The Early Window: Effects of Television on Children and Youth,* 180.

44. Ibid., 181–2.

45. Ibid., 181.

46. Ibid., 182.

47. Bill Carlino, "Operators Weigh Effects of TV Advertising Bill," *Nation's Restaurant News,* August 13, 1990, 14.

48. Policy Statement: "The Commercialization of Children's Television," American Academy of Pediatrics (July 23, 1991).

49. As quoted in Marian Burros, "A Push Is On to Fight TV Ads That Some Call Harmful to Children's Nutrition," *The New York Times,* June 12, 1991, C3.

50. Final Report: White House Conference on Food, Nutrition and Health (1969), 301.

51. Mary Story and Patricia Faulkner, "The Prime Time Diet: A Content Analysis of Eating Behavior and Food Messages in Television Program Content and Commercials," *American Journal of Public Health,* 80 (1990), 738–40.

52. Ibid., 739.

53. Ibid.

54. Lois Kaufman, "Prime-Time Nutrition," *Journal of Communication* 30, Summer 1980, 37–46.

Chapter 8: School Food

1. *Child Nutrition Program Operations Study: Second Year Report,* Office of Analysis and Evaluation, Food and Nutrition Service, U.S. Department of Agriculture, Contract No. FNS-53-3198-7-32 (June 1992).

2. John Burghardt and Barbara Devaney, "The School Nutrition Dietary Assessment Study: Summary of Findings," U.S. Department of Agriculture (October 1993).

3. "White Paper on School-Lunch Nutrition," Citizens' Commission on School Nutrition, Center for Science in the Public Interest (December 1990).

4. Mike Espy, letter included in schedule of events at "Nutrition Objectives for School Meals," hearing by the U.S. Department of Agriculture, Washington, D.C., December 7, 1993.

5. M. Patricia Snyder, Mary Story, Leslie Lytle Trenkner, "Reducing Fat and Sodium in School Lunch Programs: The LUNCHPOWER! Intervention Study," *Journal of the American Dietetic Association* 92 (1992), 1087.

6. American School Health Association et al., The National Adolescent Student Health Survey (Oakland, CA: Third Party Publishing, 1989), 99, 107.

7. Alan Meyers et al., "School Breakfast Program and School Performance," *American Journal of Diseases of Children* 143 (October 1989), 1234.

8. *Child Nutrition Programs: Issues for the 101st Congress,* Subcommittee on Elementary, Secondary, and Vocation Education, Committee on Education and Labor, House of Representatives, 100th Congress, 2nd session (December 1988), 21.

Chapter 9: Corporations Invade the Classroom

1. *What Can Be Done to Improve Nutrition Education Efforts in the Schools?* U. S. General Accounting Office (May 25, 1982), 11.

2. Barbara Shannon, Bethene Ervin, and Valerie Bernardo, "The Status of School-Based Nutrition Education in State Agencies" (Pennsylvania State University Department of Nutrition, 1990), 12.

3. Ibid., 5.

4. Joan Gussow, "Who Pays the Piper?" *Teachers College Record* (Summer 1980), 454.

5. *Selling America's Kids: Commercial Pressures on Kids of the 90's,* Consumers Union (1990), 4.

6. Sheila Harty, *The Corporate Pied Piper: Ideas for International Consumer Action on Business Propaganda in Schools,* International Organization of Consumers Unions (Malaysia, 1985), 28.

7. *Selling America's Kids,* 4.

8. "Healthy by Choice: The Minnesota Plan for Nutrition and Health," Minnesota Department of Health (December 1986), 134.

9. Student booklet, "Smart Moves for Your Health," National Dairy Council (1990), 6.

10. Laurie Petersen, "Risky Business: Marketers Make a Beeline for The Nation's Schools," *Adweek's Marketing Week,* May 14, 1990, 20.

11. Dave Wellman, "Shopping Styles of the Young and Food-Conscious," *Food & Beverage Marketing* (March 1989), 19.

12. Greg Farrell, "The Education of Joel Babbitt," *Adweek,* 4 October 1993, 26.

13. Walecia Konrad, "How Good Is Attendance in Chris Whittle's Class?" *Business Week,* January 27, 1992, 103.

14. "Risky Business," 21.

15. *Selling America's Kids,* 11.

16. "Risky Business," 21.

17. *Selling America's Kids,* 11.

18. Kerry J. Stewart et al., "Two-Year Results from FRESH: An Elementary School Nutrition Education Program for Promoting Cardiovascular Health," *Circulation Supplement I* 86 (4) (October 1992), I-144.

19. Kim Gans et al., "Heart Healthy Cook-offs in Home Economics Classes: An Evaluation with Junior High School Students," *Journal of School Health,* 60, No. 3 (March 1990), 99–102.

Chapter 10: Getting Kids to Eat Healthy Foods

1. *The Surgeon General's Report on Nutrition and Health,* Public Health Service, U.S. Department of Health and Human Services, 1988, 564.

2. Ibid., 563.

3. Judith Willis, "Good Nutrition for the Highchair Set," *FDA Consumer* (September 1985), 5.

4. *The Surgeon General's Report on Nutrition and Health,* 566–7.

5. Jukka Karjalainen et al., "A Bovine Albumin Peptide as a Possible Trigger of Insulin-Dependent Diabetes Mellitus," *New England Journal of Medicine* 327 (1992), 302–7.

6. *Pediatric Nutrition Handbook,* 2nd ed., American Academy of Pediatrics, Elk Grove Village, IL (1985), 30.

Afterword: Closing Thoughts

1. Nancy Harmon Jenkins "Voting With Your Fork," *The Boston Sunday Globe,* November 29, 1992, A17.

Index